THE MOST EFFECTIVE WAYS TO

DEFEAT CHRONIC PAIN NOW!

We dedicate this book to our patients—even those we have yet to meet—for it's you who have taught us more than we ever learned in medical school, in our residency, or in our pain fellowships. We only hope we have given as much to you as you have given to us.

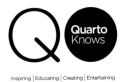

Inspiring | Educating | Creating | Entertaining

Brimming with creative inspiration, how-to projects, and useful information to enrich your everyday life, Quarto Knows is a favorite destination for those pursuing their interests and passions. Visit our site and dig deeper with our books into your area of interest: Quarto Creates, Quarto Cooks, Quarto Homes, Quarto Lives, Quarto Drives, Quarto Explores, Quarto Gifts, or Quarto Kids.

Text © 2010 Bradley S. Galer, M.D., and Charles E. Argoff, M.D.

This edition published in 2018 by Crestline,
an imprint of The Quarto Group
142 West 36th Street, 4th Floor
New York, NY 10018 USA
T (212) 779-4972 F (212) 779-6058
www.QuartoKnows.com

First published in the USA in 2010 by Fair Winds Press,
an imprint of The Quarto Group, 100 Cummings Center,
Suite 265D, Beverly, MA 01915-6101

10 9 8 7 6 5 4 3 2 1

Crestline titles are also available at discount for retail, wholesale, promotional, and bulk purchase. For details, contact the Special Sales Manager by email at specialsales@quarto.com or by mail at The Quarto Group, Attn: Special Sales Manager, 401 Second Avenue North, Suite 310, Minneapolis, MN 55401, USA.

ISBN-13: 978-0-7858-3591-2

Printed and bound in China

Book design: Kathie Alexander
Layout: Kathie Alexander
Illustrations: Robert Brandt
Page 23: @ Universal Images Group Limited/Alamy
Page 25, 149, and 192: ZEPHYR/Science Photo Library
Page 56: © Scott Camazine/Alamy
Page 67: © Science Photo Library/Alamy

The information in this book is for educational purposes only.
It is not intended to replace the advice of a physician or medical practitioner.
Please see your health-care provider before beginning any new health program.

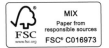

THE MOST EFFECTIVE WAYS TO

DEFEAT CHRONIC PAIN NOW!

BRADLEY S. GALER, M.D.

Co-founder of American Academy of Neurology Pain Medicine Special Interest
Group, Named one of the leading doctors in pain management
by the Best Doctors in America

CHARLES E. ARGOFF, M.D.

Co-founder of American Academy of Neurology Pain Medicine
Special Interest Group. Professor of Neurology, Albany Medical College;
Director, Comprehensive Pain Program, Albany Medical Center

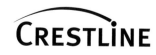

CONTENTS

3 | Understanding Your Pain / **217**

Introduction: A Silent Pandemic

Chronic pain is a silent pandemic, affecting people all over the world, regardless of age, ethnicity, or race. It is a condition that acknowledges no boundaries. Chronic pain is one of the most common medical problems, especially among those of us who are approaching "middle age"! We bet that if you ask anyone you know— whether at work, in your church, or at your child's Little League game—you will find that he or she either suffers from chronic pain or has a family member or good friend who does. Everyone knows someone who suffers from chronic pain.

It has been estimated that about one-third of all Americans suffer from chronic pain. That means about 105 million people in the United States are living with conditions including chronic back and neck pain and migraine headaches. A study published in 2003 found that approximately 150 million Americans took medications—including both prescription and over-the-counter drugs—during the previous months to relieve their acute and/or chronic pain.

As our population ages, these numbers are going to increase. Indeed, chronic pain is a bigger health problem than most other medical conditions that get more "airplay." Because you cannot see it, chronic pain is easy to ignore and discount; because it attracts less attention, it receives less government funding for research. Insurance companies compound this problem by frequently denying appropriate medical care for chronic pain sufferers—and that's a shame.

Another unbelievable and scary fact is that most doctors are not properly educated in the management of chronic pain. Pain courses are rarely if ever taught in medical schools. During their years of internship training and residency, doctors are seldom instructed in how to properly diagnose and treat chronic pain. And who suffers as a result of this lack of education? You do.

Since the mid-1980s, during our last years in medical school, we have devoted our careers to helping people who are suffering from chronic pain (in fact, that's how we met and became friends and colleagues). We have been blessed to learn from pain experts worldwide and privileged to work alongside some of the best pain management providers of all time. Indeed, we were lucky enough to be trained by and work with the "Hall of Famers" of pain management.

However, we have also witnessed far too much bad pain management over the past twenty-plus years, and we feel it is our obligation to help anyone who will listen. That's why we combined our knowledge and experience to write this book, a personal "survival guide" for chronic pain sufferers. Our aim is to present all the important facts—the good, the bad, and the ugly. We want to give you real answers to your tough questions.

Many of you may be given the wrong advice by undereducated or selfish doctors and other professionals, or be prescribed the wrong medication or treatment based on overzealous pharmaceutical, supplement, or device companies. Many of you face roadblocks to obtaining appropriate care from your insurance companies. This is unacceptable—you are already suffering enough!

You don't have to fall victim to the uninformed doctors, insurance companies, workers' compensation systems, drug companies, and device makers who all want to make a buck either by selling you a "cure" or by making recommendations based on their narrow worldview about chronic pain. You need to empower yourself with knowledge about your disease so that you know more than these "deciders," most of whom are not truly educated on the subject of chronic pain. If we can spare you more pain and suffering by teaching you all there is to know about your pain—and warn you about what and whom to look out for—we will have done our duty as pain management doctors.

To that end, we've written in layman's language as much as possible throughout the book, particularly in Part 1, which addresses the specific pain conditions in detail. Why? Because this book is our offering to you—the patient. You are the one living with chronic pain, and it is your right to have the information you need—in a way that you can easily understand—so you can be an active participant in resolving it. Start with Part 1, where you'll find chapters covering specific types of pain. We'll tell you what treatments have been shown to work and highlight the most cutting-edge developments. In Part 2, we'll cover treatments and therapies in much more detail—and with a bit more medical-speak, but don't worry, this important information is also written to serve you, the patient, the ultimate "decider" of care. Finally, don't skip Part 3! We discuss what pain is, why we all have pain, how one experiences it, how factors like stress affect it, and how your nervous system works. While there may be a few sections that bring back unpleasant memories of high school biology, this section teaches you (in easy-to-understand words) the key basics behind how pain works in the body. Again, our aim is to help you by giving you in "plain English" the most important information about pain that we have learned over our multiple decades of being pain doctors.

This book is not intended to replace the services of a physician. Any application of the recommendations set forth is at the reader's discretion. As every person's medical condition is unique, the reader should consult with his or her own physician or specialist concerning the recommendations in this book.

We wish you all the best, and hope you find some pain relief and start enjoying life again.

PART 1

Recognize and Relieve Your Chronic Pain

CHAPTER 1

Beating Your Back Pain

Myofascial dysfunction is the most common—

and most misdiagnosed—culprit.

the PRESCRIPTION for BACK PAIN

Although most people fear they have a herniated (bulging) disc that will require surgery, the majority of back pain sufferers do not have a herniated disc, and even if they do they do not need surgery.

Thus, the first prescription we write to you is to avoid initially seeing a back surgeon who may recommend that you go "under the knife." Also, avoid first seeing a pain management doctor who only specializes in nerve blocks, because he or she will probably recommend repeated epidural nerve blocks that have very questionable efficacy.

The most common culprit in back pain is usually deep, chronic muscle spasms (myofascial dysfunction), which surgery cannot help. The best prescription, then, is multimodal therapy such as active physical therapy (PT) combined with medications for pain that can keep you on track with the physical program. "Nontraditional" treatments such as acupuncture and yoga also can help.

- ✓ Medications for pain
- ✓ Active PT
- ✓ Therapeutic massage
- ✓ Acupuncture
- ✓ Yoga

"Invisible" Back Pain: A Patient's Story

I have had back pain for two years now. Initially, I had back surgery one month after I injured my back lifting a heavy box at work. The surgeon said I had a "bulging disc" that was the cause of my pain and performed a discectomy on me almost eighteen months ago, removing part of my herniated disc in my back that was seen on a magnetic resonance imaging (MRI) scan. He said the surgery was a success. Well, maybe for him, but not for me! I have continued to have severe back pain. In fact, it's worse now than before the surgery. Many back surgeon specialists have examined me and looked at all the tests I've had both before and after the surgery—computed tomography (CT) scans, MRIs, electromyographies (EMGs), bone scans, and God knows what else. The tests have been normal, or the doctors say they see "what you expect to see after back surgery," so now I don't know what to think. The experts say they can't see why I have pain; is it all in my head?

Symptoms of Back Pain

You have back pain, which, for many people, stays mainly in the region of the lower back. However, your pain may spread to your buttocks, hips, and legs. Most people describe their pain as "aching" and "deep." Some describe it as "burning" or "sharp." If you have pain, you may feel it "shooting" and "radiating" into your legs.

Most people with back pain have very tight and tender muscles in their lower back. When muscles are in chronic spasm, they often cause pain not only where the muscles are located, but also in other areas of the body, beyond the location of the muscles. This is called *referred pain*. With low-back myofascial pain, the referred pain can be felt in your butt, in your hips, down your leg, and into your foot, but most folks don't have referred pain in all of these body regions.

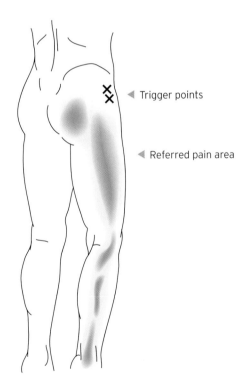

◀ Trigger points

◀ Referred pain area

TRIGGER POINTS MAY CAUSE SHOOTING PAIN

Tight, tender muscles in spasm may also have tight knots called *myofascial trigger points*, which can also cause referred pain. Trigger points in your lower back can cause you to feel pain in your hip and buttock, or cause a shooting pain down into your leg. Most doctors are taught that a pain in one leg and foot is caused by sciatica, a nerve that forms near the lower spine that is being pinched by a swollen disc, so most will automatically assume this is the diagnosis. Thus, you can understand how doctors who aren't trained in myofascial back pain and don't examine you for this condition will misdiagnose you with a bulging disc and squeezed nerve. Unfortunately, this happens perhaps as often as ninety out of 100 times, even if the patient is evaluated by a good neurologist or back surgeon. Believe it or not, they just don't know!

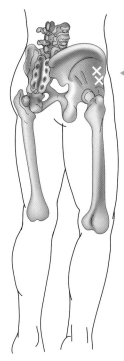

◀ Trigger points in the muscles of the hip (gluteus minimus) can cause radiating pain in the buttock and down the leg

Trigger Points Develop When the Sarcomeres Get Stuck

To understand what trigger points are and why they can develop, first you have to understand what makes a muscle contract. The part of the muscle fiber that contracts is the sarcomere, which is microscopic in size. Each muscle contains millions of sarcomeres. When the sarcomeres within a muscle join together in unison, similar to when you interlock your fingers, the muscle will contract. A trigger point develops in a muscle when the sarcomeres become injured or are overstimulated from overuse; this causes a chemical imbalance that prohibits the sarcomeres from unlocking from their interlocked state. (This is still a scientific hypothesis, and is not yet conclusively proven.)

Who Gets Chronic Back Pain?

As you might imagine, a lot of research has gone into trying to answer this question. What the research found might surprise you (as it has many doctors, patients, and employers): There are no biological risk factors (e.g., being obese, having bad posture, etc.) for developing chronic back pain after an injury at work. Unless you have had a significant herniated disc or a piece of your disc in your spinal canal has broken off and is floating in your spinal fluid (which is very rare), back injuries that seemingly cause mild to moderate disc bulge do not necessarily cause chronic low back pain.

Even more surprising, no particular type of jobs, such as lifting heavy objects, make an individual more likely to develop back pain. Although you may have nagging back pain that comes and goes if you sit too long in your office chair (which will not happen if you take breaks to do some stretching exercises!), you will not develop chronic debilitating back pain unless you have a certain significant risk factor!

(continued)

Back Pain is a Common Problem

Back pain is almost as widespread as the common cold. Studies have shown that each of us has about a 75 percent chance of experiencing back pain sometime during our life. This chapter will help you not only if you have back pain now, but also prepare all of us for the future and assist any loved ones who are currently suffering from this condition. In this book, we will be talking mostly about chronic back pain that has lasted for several months and is located in the lumbar region, the lowest part of your back.

As we said, the most common cause of this pain is chronic muscle spasm, also called *myofascial dysfunction*. We have all had acute muscle spasms, in which a muscle spontaneously contracts or cramps, causing sharp, burning, stabbing, and/or aching pain at the site of the spasm. Myofascial dysfunction occurs when a muscle or group of muscles (as well as ligaments and tendons) becomes disposed to suddenly going into a spasm or cramp chronically. There may be times when the muscle is relaxed, but at any time it may become dysfunctional and go into a spasm or cramping mode.

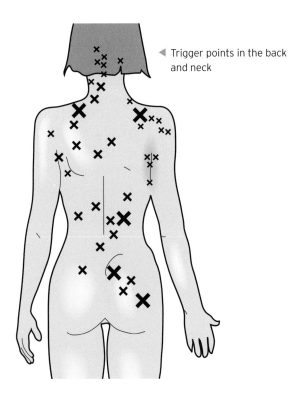

◄ Trigger points in the back and neck

All soft tissues (muscles, ligaments, and tendons) can go into a chronic state of hypersensitivity to spasm and cramping due to injury or trauma, surgery, or repetitive use, disuse, or misuse. Like lots of our body parts, we take our muscles, ligaments, and tendons for granted; if we use them too much or too little, they can go into an abnormal state and seemingly protest their misuse! Luckily, though, once we learn how to use them properly, the muscles can easily go back into their happy, nonpainful state.

Medications to Treat Back Pain

Although no drug truly acts to relieve the muscle spasm at the source of most folks' back pain, many different types of medications can alleviate the pain you feel. Medications can improve your quality of life and optimize the effects of PT. There really isn't a "most-effective" medication; rather, your doctor should prescribe the drugs on a trial-and-error basis, first using the ones with the least number of possible side effects (more on this in chapter 8).

NSAIDS AND COX-2 INHIBITORS REDUCE INFLAMMATION

At times, patients do find relief from the anti-inflammatory and general pain-relieving effects of nonsteroidal anti-inflammatory drugs (NSAIDs, such as Voltaren, Motrin, and Aleve) and COX-2 inhibitor medications (Celebrex) when taken orally as pills, tablets, and capsules. However, these usually offer only slight to moderate relief at best. Also, these medications can cause potentially serious side effects if consumed too frequently or at too high a dose, even if bought as over-the-counter (OTC) preparations. If taken incorrectly, they can cause serious liver, kidney, and heart problems. However, if taken as recommended, these medications can be useful for many people. For more information on how they work, see "Medications to Treat OA Pain," page 49.

If one of these medications doesn't give you enough relief or gives you intolerable side effects—the most common being upset stomach—it's worthwhile to try a few others to find one that does give you meaningful pain relief without bad side effects, as everyone will react differently to each.

(Who Gets Chronic Back Pain? continued)

The factor that has been identified to put people at risk for developing chronic back pain is a lack of satisfaction and control over one's job. The work-related injury doesn't even have to be severe; the pain can be caused by a minor twisting of the back or by lifting a few books or reams of paper.

In other words, if you are not happy in your job and you feel like your boss is a micromanaging jerk, or you don't feel valued for the work you do, you may be at risk for developing chronic back pain. Sadly, some research shows that many if not most people are not happy or satisfied in their jobs, which may explain why the condition is so common! And especially with the current economy the way it has been, more and more people will be taking jobs they do not find satisfying and will be at risk for developing chronic low back pain.

TOPICAL NSAIDS HAVE FEWER SIDE EFFECTS

In the United States, topical NSAID preparations such as Pennsaid, Voltaren Gel, and Flector Patch have recently been FDA-approved for treating certain chronic pain conditions such as arthritis and acute sports injury pain. Although they have not been tested to treat chronic musculoskeletal pain, it is likely that these lotions, creams, and patches may produce similar pain relief as the same drug taken orally, but with less chance of developing the side effects associated with ingesting pills or capsules. These types of drugs, available in Europe and Asia for several decades, have the same medicine found in oral NSAIDs, but produce lower amounts of the drug in the blood because they act locally, and thus theoretically reduce the risks for serious and bothersome side effects.

For topical NSAIDs, the recommended application for Pennsaid and Voltaren Gel is four times per day directly to the site of pain. The recommended dose for the Flector Patch, a topical NSAID, is one patch every twelve hours.

THE LIDOCAINE PATCH 5% (LIDODERM) REDUCES PAIN

Although the lidocaine patch is not FDA-approved to treat back pain, several published studies have shown that some patients with back pain report very good relief and no serious side effects from applying up to four lidocaine patches directly to their lower back region. (Lidoderm is only FDA-approved to treat chronic nerve pain after shingles, a condition called *postherpetic neuralgia*.)

The FDA-approved dosing for lidocaine patch 5% is up to three patches at a time applied to the painful area for twelve hours on and then twelve hours off. However, many studies have been published showing that it is safe to use up to four patches at a time, keeping them on for twenty-four hours and then putting on new patches.

TRAMADOL COMBINES TWO MECHANISMS

Tramadol is an interesting drug with several different pain-relieving mechanisms, including acting as a weak opioid (sometimes called *narcotic*) combined with the ability to work on the chemicals norepinephrine and serotonin that have been shown to help produce pain relief in the spinal cord and brain. Several good studies show that some patients with back pain experience significant pain relief with tramadol and without intolerable side effects. Tramadol is now available both as a long-acting once-per-day pill (Ryzolt and Ultram ER) as well as immediate-release pills taken four times per day (Ultram and generics). One available preparation of tramadol is combined with acetaminophen (Ultracet).

DULOXETINE (CYMBALTA) WORKS IN THE SPINE AND BRAIN

Recently, scientific trials have shown that duloxetine can produce very good pain relief in patients with back pain. Duloxetine works on two neurotransmitter chemicals involved in the perception of pain in the spinal cord and brain, norepinephrine and serotonin. It is available as a pill and is most often taken once daily.

OPIOIDS ARE CAUTIOUSLY RECOMMENDED FOR CERTAIN PATIENTS

Opioid medication (narcotics) has recently been shown to be of benefit for some people suffering from moderate to severe back pain. Like all medications used in treating back pain, opioids are not a cure, but when prescribed appropriately they can improve the chances of an active PT program being successful.

In our opinion, opioids should not routinely be prescribed as first-line medication for many patients with back pain because of their potential for side effects, the rare risk of addiction, and the potential for misuse and diversion (someone taking your pills for a high or to sell for money) of these types of medications. However, for some patients, opioid medication can significantly increase quality of life and can mean the difference between success and failure with the needed PT program. It is vital that you use all medications as prescribed to maximize both their pain relieving benefit as well as your safety.

What's New: FDA Approvals for Back Pain

Tapentadol (marketed as Nucynta), like tramadol, acts on two chemicals in the spinal cord and brain: the opiate system and the neurochemical norepinephrine, both neurotransmitters that we naturally have in our body that have been shown to be involved in our natural pain-relieving pathways. Tapentadol has been shown in studies to relieve low back pain and other types of chronic pain (and acute pain). It is currently available only as a short-acting, immediate-release pill, but an extended-release pill is under development.

Tanezumab is being developed by the pharmaceutical company Pfizer to treat multiple types of chronic pain. This is truly a novel type of drug, as it works to block the protein nerve growth factor that plays a big part in the development of pain after injury and inflammation. As this book went to press, tanezumab had a major setback as the FDA raised concerns about the potential safety of this drug, especially in patients with osteoarthritis. If it eventually receives FDA approval, patients will likely be required to inject tanezumab every eight to twelve weeks for treatment to be successful.

⚡ Back Alert!

Work Through the Initial Pain

With successful active PT, it is expected that pain may get slightly worse during the initial phases before it gets better. This is because the muscles at the core of your problem have gotten used to being in a spastic state, so initially, moving them can cause them to go into further spasm, and hence can cause more pain. However, you should realize that in fact, this initial worsening of your pain is a good sign because it means the muscles responsible for your back pain are the ones receiving the needed treatment.

We've seen too many patients use pain as their guide for daily activity levels. That is, on the "good days" they overdo it, and on the "bad days" they become couch potatoes. Let's say Monday and Tuesday were bad pain days, so you stayed in bed or on the couch for most of the day. Wednesday was a nice, sunny day and your pain was better, so you tried to accomplish two days' worth of activities to make up for lost time. And then guess what? On Thursday, you were back in bed and on the couch. Does this sound familiar? This isn't sensible!

(continued)

Nonmedication Therapies for Back Pain Relief

We strongly believe these are more important than medication therapy (or injections, devices, or surgery) for the vast majority of people with back pain. The following types of therapies aim to reduce the chronic muscle spasms and tight/tender ligaments and tendons associated with back pain, and are crucial in alleviating the symptoms related to this condition.

If you suffer from this all-too-common medical problem, you should find an experienced pain practitioner who can perform one of these therapies (or a mixture) to target the crux of your problem and truly resolve your spasms and back pain. And remember, just because a doctor has "Pain Management" next to his or her name does not mean he or she knows how to appropriately evaluate and treat back pain. The old saying "If all you have is a hammer, everything looks like a nail" is true with doctors too; a back surgeon is most likely to recommend back surgery and an interventional pain management specialist is most likely to recommend nerve blocks whether you truly need them or not.

ACTIVE PHYSICAL THERAPY (PT) IS PARAMOUNT

All pain management experts agree that an active PT program is the most important treatment for patients with back pain that is not due to disc disease. This generally refers to a program that involves the patient gradually increasing the use of relevant muscles through stretching, strengthening, and endurance exercises. Your program will enable you to gradually increase how often and for what length of time you can use the muscles that are causing your back pain.

It is very important that patients with back pain work with a physical therapist who has been trained to treat this condition. Too often, untrained physical therapists will treat all back pain patients the same way, which is with "passive" modalities such as massage, heat packs, and ultrasound, resulting in inappropriate treatment and suboptimal results. By identifying the exact muscles at the core of your back pain, the physical therapist can design a tailored exercise and therapeutic program that takes direct aim at your underlying problem.

ACUPUNCTURE IS SAFE AND MAY BE BENEFICIAL

Many back pain patients report significant pain relief with a series of acupuncture treatments performed by a trained acupuncturist. Though scientific studies have shown mixed results (both positive and negative) with this form of therapy, it is our opinion that acupuncture can be a safe and potentially very helpful treatment for enough back pain patients that it may be considered.

TRIGGER-POINT INJECTIONS RELEASE THE KNOTS

Trigger-point injections (TPIs) are just what the name implies: injections made directly into the tight, spastic region of the muscle. TPIs can be done via several different techniques, including just inserting an acupuncture needle (also called *dry-needling*), injecting lidocaine or another local anesthetic drug, injecting a steroid, or injecting a local anesthetic with a steroid (see chapter 9). In our view, there is no real advantage to injecting any drug into the trigger point (except perhaps botulinum toxin, also known as BOTOX, MYBLOC or DYSPORT); however, some patients claim they experience less pain and discomfort with the acute pain associated with TPI if lidocaine or another local anesthetic is injected into the trigger point. TPIs can work for days, weeks, or even months to alleviate pain and increase movement.

It is not clear how often TPIs should be given. Most pain doctors recommend an initial trial of weekly TPIs for four to six weeks, and then reassessing to see if the patient is experiencing a positive outcome. Again, it is critically important that during this TPI trial, the patient is also enrolled in an active PT program.

HEAT TREATMENT OFFERS SHORT-TERM RELIEF

Over the past several years, we have seen a marketing push to treat all types of pain, including back pain, with an applied heat wrap (e.g., the OTC heat wrap ThermaCare). There is some evidence that heat-wrap therapy can provide a small degree of short-term pain relief in patients with back pain.

A similar treatment for back pain is the application of a focused heat source directly at the myofascial trigger points; this is referred to as *focal heat trigger-point (FHTP) therapy*. This treatment acts like a TPI, but is not invasive and the patient can do it at home.

One such FHTP device, Zeno, is an OTC treatment for acne that we've used to provide TPIs with some success.

(Back Alert! continued)

You should be doing the same amount of activity and exercise every day, regardless of your pain level. For instance, if you have not been active at all for several months, you should start small—say, two to five minutes of gentle exercise per day. Then every seven to fourteen days, gradually increase the amount of exercise by 5 percent to 10 percent, again regardless of your pain level. The key message is to take it "slow and steady," and not to base your level of daily activity and exercise on the amount of pain you are feeling that day.

Back Alert!

Drawbacks to TPIs The first few TPIs you receive can be quite painful. The muscle may actually go into deeper spasms before it eventually relearns how to relax. The key with myofascial TPIs is that the patient simultaneously engages in an active PT program. Despite potential drawbacks, patients with back pain should seriously consider TPIs from an experienced physician as a safe treatment to help relieve the symptoms of their condition.

CRANIOSACRAL THERAPY WORKS FOR SOME

Some patients with myofascial pain report significant pain relief and improved function with craniosacral therapy. These types of treatments should be performed by trained therapists with experience in treating patients with chronic pain.

THERAPEUTIC MASSAGE AND ACUPRESSURE MAY ALSO WORK

Some evidence suggests that therapeutic massage and acupressure therapy may prove beneficial in some patients with back pain. Again, these therapies should be paired with an active PT/exercise program. Also, it is important not to just get a great body massage at your local spa, but instead to find a therapeutic massage therapist who knows how to treat back pain.

GENTLE YOGA INCREASES STRENGTH AND FLEXIBILITY

There are many different types of yoga, some gentle and others more demanding. The back pain sufferer should find a gentle type of yoga, such as hatha yoga. Hatha yoga is a slow-paced stretching class with some simple breathing exercises and meditations usually done in a seated position. A recent study of yoga and chronic back pain found that after twelve weeks of yoga, 73 percent of the yoga group said they had overall improvement in back pain, as compared with 27 percent of the control group that continued to see their doctor and take their recommended treatments.

CHIROPRACTORS ARE CAUTIOUSLY RECOMMENDED

Although chiropractic treatments are one of the more common treatments people seek when they have back pain, we have to warn you that we only cautiously recommend such treatment. Studies have shown that chiropractic manipulations can help improve the symptoms of back pain, but there is a potential risk of serious injury if you don't have a "normal" back (see sidebar "Before You See a Chiropractor"). As with any health care practitioner treating your condition, it is important that the chiropractor be well experienced in treating chronic back pain.

Chiropractic medicine is based on the belief that the spine may have restricted movement that leads to pain and poor function. When a chiropractor "manipulates" your back (also called *spinal adjustment*), he or she will apply a sudden force to your back bones, pushing or pulling the vertebrae to different unnatural positions. This application of force is what causes the popping and cracking sounds you hear emanating from their offices! At times, a chiropractor may also use massage and gentle stretching techniques as well.

STRESS MANAGEMENT TECHNIQUES REDUCE TENSION

As we discuss in chapter 17, the stress reaction has been shown to cause worsening muscle spasms, especially in muscles that are prone to spasm (myofascial dysfunction). Therefore, it makes sense that stress management techniques, such as relaxation, imagery, and biofeedback, can all play a very important role in the treatment of back pain.

PSYCHOLOGICAL TREATMENTS RELIEVE THE MIND AND BACK

Many back pain patients develop depression due to their constant, unrelenting, debilitating pain. If this happens to you, you should seek psychological treatment. Studies have shown that patients with all types of chronic pain and depression or anxiety will be less responsive to their pain treatments if these psychiatric conditions are not also treated. Back pain patients who may have a psychiatric condition, such as depression, anxiety, or post-traumatic stress disorder, should be evaluated by a psychiatrist or psychologist. Depending on the severity of your condition, he or she may recommend a simple course of antidepressant medication and/or other types of psychological therapies, such as cognitive-behavioral therapy (see chapter 11).

Feeling Depressed Is Par for the Course

Don't be ashamed if you have one of these psychological conditions because of your back pain. Almost every patient we have treated with chronic back pain has at some point during his or her illness developed depression or another psychological condition because of how his or her life has been negatively affected by their back pain.

Back Alert!

Before You See a Chiropractor
It is very important that your diagnosis of myofascial back pain be made by a trained back pain physician before you see a chiropractor. If your back pain is actually coming from true disc disease, some of the chiropractic manipulations performed could result in serious neurological damage.

Back Alert!

No Case for Nerve Blocks

We believe there is no role for a series of nerve blocks in the treatment of chronic back pain unless it is clear that the cause of your chronic back pain has been shown to be responsive to nerve blocks. Most commonly, "being responsive" means providing a noticeable degree of pain relief for a period of weeks to months. Proceed cautiously if you are promised 100 percent pain relief forever! We've seen too many patients go to nerve block shops (doctors and clinics that treat all forms of pain with only nerve blocks) and receive dozens of injections without any long-term good results, only to stop these treatments with no change in their pain but with a much lighter wallet. **Beware of "pain doctors" who only know how to treat pain with a sharp needle aimed for your back!**

Therapies That Do Not Work For Back Pain

"MUSCLE RELAXANTS" ARE REALLY SEDATIVES

Though many drugs have been marketed as "muscle relaxants," they do not actually relax the muscles! In fact, no drug has been shown to significantly reduce the spasm of chronic myofascial pain conditions. Rather, muscle relaxer drugs likely work similarly to Valium and "relax" your muscles only by sedating you. When you're asleep, you naturally relax your muscles—but you can't live in a sedated state your whole life, despite what that catchy Ramones song says!

PASSIVE PT FEELS GOOD ONLY BRIEFLY

Many—if not most—physical therapists are trained in only passive, "feel good" therapies, such as warm baths, gentle massage, and ultrasound. Ultrasound is a technique in which sound waves are applied to the muscles of your back in hopes of getting them to relax. Although these types of PT techniques feel great when you get them, they will not treat, resolve, or cure your back problem.

SURGERY IS NOT WARRANTED FOR BACK PAIN FROM SPASMS

There is absolutely no role for surgery in the treatment of chronic back pain due to muscle spasm. We have seen far too many patients with back pain who want a quick fix and hope to find a surgeon who is willing to do back surgery on them. **Not only does this not help, but often it makes the pain and disability worse.** Please don't be one of these folks!

SPINAL CORD STIMULATION IS A COSTLY LAST RESORT

Although evidence suggests that spinal cord stimulation may be of benefit to some patients with various types of back pain, it is our opinion that this expensive type of treatment should most often be reserved as a last resort for patients with back pain. Here, too, beware of pain specialists who most often only insert spinal cord stimulators for all sorts of pain. **Some of these doctors accumulate a great deal of wealth from these procedures, so they are quick to recommend this type of treatment.**

Diagnosing Back Pain

First, to diagnose the cause of your back pain, you'll need to have a neurologist, a physical medicine/rehabilitation doctor, or a properly-trained primary care doctor evaluate you. These types of doctors are specialists in the examination of the nerves in your spine, and thus can assess your back for any potential associated neurological abnormalities. As with most patients with back pain, your neurological examination will likely be normal (if not, see the Back Alert! about warning signs).

Second, upon completing a myofascial examination, the doctor will likely find muscle trigger points that reproduce your pain when palpated and gently pressed. That's it; no "fancy-schmancy" expensive tests needed!

Back Alert!

Unwarranted Surgeries Cause Problems When we were young pain doctors and patients came to us after back surgery still in pain, we thought we were seeing only a biased sample; that maybe there were many successful back surgeries and we were seeing only the people who did not do well. Unfortunately, that does not appear to be the case. Too many folks are advised to undergo back surgery when they don't need it, and many of them are getting surgeries, such as fusions, that produce a host of new problems that are difficult if not impossible to treat without more surgery. Beware!

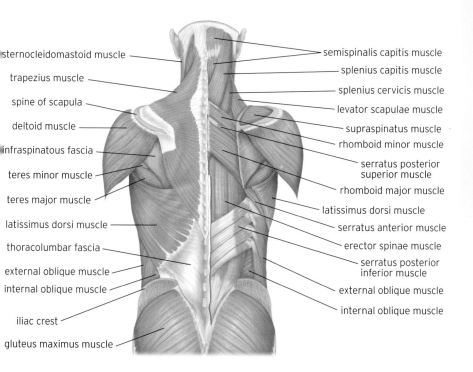

sternocleidomastoid muscle
trapezius muscle
spine of scapula
deltoid muscle
infraspinatous fascia
teres minor muscle
teres major muscle
latissimus dorsi muscle
thoracolumbar fascia
external oblique muscle
internal oblique muscle
iliac crest
gluteus maximus muscle

semispinalis capitis muscle
splenius capitis muscle
splenius cervicis muscle
levator scapulae muscle
supraspinatus muscle
rhomboid minor muscle
serratus posterior superior muscle
rhomboid major muscle
latissimus dorsi muscle
serratus anterior muscle
erector spinae muscle
serratus posterior inferior muscle
external oblique muscle
internal oblique muscle

▲ The back has many muscles, all of which may have trigger points

23

⚡ Examination Findings: Back Pain

The neurological examination in patients with back pain due to muscle spasm is completely normal. However, definite abnormalities are found on the myofascial examination of the muscles of the lower back. When the doctor assesses the muscles for trigger points, he or she will find that lightly pushing on the tight and tender muscles will be painful and can mimic the patient's pain symptoms. Quite often, gently pushing on these tight muscles will cause the patient's pain to spread (e.g., into the buttock and down into the leg).

FINDING MYOFASCIAL TRIGGER POINTS

Although diagnosing myofascial trigger points is not rocket science, unfortunately most doctors aren't trained to perform a proper evaluation for trigger points, and may not even be aware of what a trigger point is.

To find a myofascial trigger point, a doctor should gently rub his or her fingers along your muscles, ligaments, and tendons and feel for tight, hard knots, and then gently and slowly push these tight knots with his or her thumb to see your reaction. We all have trigger points at different times. To make a diagnosis of myofascial back pain, the trigger points in your back region, when pressed, should cause you to have a certain reaction.

First, myofascial trigger points responsible for your pain may cause what's called a *twitch response*, meaning the doctor can feel the muscle, tendon, or ligament actually twitch. Second, you will feel pain that mimics the pain you feel spontaneously. Third, you may also feel referred pain, so you will feel pain not only where the doctor is pressing, but also in a different location. For instance, trigger points in muscles along the lower back region can cause you to feel pain in your hip, buttock, and even leg.

Because doctors aren't often trained in trigger points, they mistakenly diagnose pain that starts in the back and shoots into your buttock or leg as "sciatica," caused by a bulging disc that is irritating or squeezing a nerve root coming out of your spine. That's why it's critically important that you be examined by an experienced and knowledgeable doctor.

NO LAB TESTS NEEDED TO DIAGNOSE MOST BACK PAIN

Radiology tests, such as X-rays, CT scans, and MRIs, do not provide the cause for the vast majority of patients with back pain. Interestingly, however, a recent study from Stanford University showed that areas of the United States with the highest number of MRIs also have the highest number of surgeries for low back pain, with the senior scientist concluding, "The net result is increased risks of unnecessary surgery for patients and increased costs for everybody else."

Electromyograms (EMG) and nerve conduction (NCV) tests may or may not demonstrate abnormal muscle spasm, but they do not show any nerve damage. EMG/NCV tests are most often completely normal in persons with back pain.

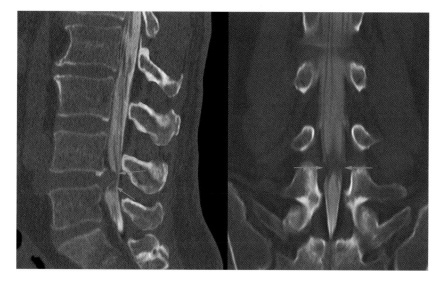

▲ Slipped Disc/Disc Bulge, commonly misunderstood

What to Expect from a Neurological Examination

For all chronic pain conditions, your doctor should perform a thorough neurological examination, which has three basic parts:

Motor: The doctor will have you push and pull your different muscles to evaluate their strength.

Sensory: The doctor will test your sensory perception as various objects touch your body; each object evaluates different nerves and parts of your nervous system. These include lightly rubbing a finger or a Q-tip across your skin, poking you with a pin (you should say "ouch"), and placing a vibrating tuning fork on your toe and finger joints, and asking if you feel a vibration.

Reflexes: The doctor will take out his or her trusty reflex hammer and check your reflexes not only at your knee, but also at your ankles, elbow, and wrist.

Less Common Causes of Back Pain

Although by far the most common cause of chronic back pain is muscle spasm and most people are most fearful of having a herniated disc, there are other less common problems you should be aware of:

SPONDYLOLISTHESIS

What is it? Spondylolisthesis occurs when the vertebral bone in the lower part of the spine slips forward and onto the vertebra below it.

Diagnosis:
- Diagnosis is easily made via a simple plain X-ray of the lower back.

Symptoms:
- Pain is felt in the lower back, and possibly in the buttocks and hips.
- The back feels stiff.
- Tenderness is felt in the region of the slipped vertebra.

Treatment:
- For most patients, the treatment is similar to that for myofascial back pain.
- Patients with severe pain or severe slippage that does not respond to conservative treatment may require surgery to fuse the vertebral bones together.

SPINAL STENOSIS

What is it? Spinal stenosis is a narrowing of the central canal (hole) in which the spine nerves travel.

Diagnosis:
- On examination, patients with lumbar (low back) stenosis often have weakness and some abnormal sensations in their legs, which they may not even notice. Patients with cervical (neck) stenosis have weakness and abnormal sensations in their arms, hands, or fingers.
- Laboratory tests such as MRI/CT scans and plain X-rays show narrowing of the spinal canal.
- EMG may also help make the diagnosis.

Symptoms:
For lower back spinal stenosis:
- Commonly, patients complain of pain or cramping in their legs with prolonged standing or walking, which quickly improves with bending over or sitting down.
- Pain may spread into the legs.
- Patients may experience numbness and tingling in the legs.

For neck spinal stenosis:
- Patients experience pain and cramping in the shoulders, arms, and legs.
- The hands are clumsy.
- Sometimes trouble walking and bad balance can also occur.

Treatment:
This condition is much more common in the low back than in the neck region

- Again, all patients should initially try nonsurgical therapies for at least three months, including active PT and medication.
- If conservative therapy fails, epidural nerve blocks may be tried prior to surgery.
- As a last resort, surgery may be needed to increase the opening where the disease process has narrowed the canal.

ANKYLOSING SPONDYLITIS

What is it? This is a chronic inflammatory arthritis and auto-immune condition that eventually may cause abnormal spine and pelvis bone growth and fusion of the bones. This condition is much more common in the low back than in the neck region. It is believed to be an inherited genetic disorder.

Diagnosis:
- In later stages, plain X-rays and MRI/CT scans can show abnormalities.
- Blood tests can be helpful to demonstrate an abnormal inflammatory process, such as erythrocyte sedimentation rate and C-reactive protein (CRP).
- Genetic testing for the HLA-B27 gene can also be used to diagnose this condition.

Symptoms:
- In early stages, this condition may mimic myofascial back pain.
- As the disease progresses, symptoms spread to possibly include stiffness of the entire spine and an inability to take deep breaths (rib involvement).
- A telltale sign is if you develop eye pain or blurred vision, as the eye may become involved in the disease process.
- When A.S. involves the neck, which is not common, symptoms include neck pain and stiffness with loss of neck movement.

Treatment:
Here is where specific medications can have a significant effect on the disease process. These drugs include:
- NSAIDs, as described in chapter 8.
- Disease-modifying antirheumatic drugs, such as sulfasalazine or methotrexate. These may help to limit the inflammation and damage. However, there are potential serious side effects of low blood counts and liver damage that need to be monitored during treatment with these drugs.
- Corticosteroids. When prescribed chronically, these may also help to reduce the inflammatory process and minimize damage in severe cases, as back pain is one of the rare conditions in which the benefits of chronic steroid use may outweigh the risks.
- Tumor necrosis factor blockers, such as adalimumab (Humira), etanercept (Enbrel), and infliximab (Remicade). These are relatively new types of drugs that block a specific protein responsible for inflammation. These drugs can all have fairly dramatic positive results, but also have the potential for very serious side effects, including infections such as tuberculosis, seizures, or inflammation of the nerves of the eyes, worsening of heart failure, a lupus-like syndrome, and lymphoma, a type of cancer.

Get the Facts: MRI/CT Scans and Back Pain

Here are some important facts you and your doctor should know about MRI/CT scans and back pain (and actually this applies to most chronic pain conditions):

Fact 1: Disc bulges happen naturally, often with no pain. Many studies have demonstrated that most people who have disc bulges (herniated discs) on CT/MRI scans actually have no back pain. It has been shown that when people reach middle age, more than half of those who have MRI/CT scans show bulging discs but have absolutely no pain. Therefore, a bulging disc is not automatically the reason for your pain. Bulging discs are now considered a natural part of the aging process.

Fact 2: Disc bulges can get better if left alone. Several studies have shown that the natural course of a bulging, herniated disc (if left alone) is that it repairs itself! Over several months, the disc gradually goes back to where it belongs.

(continued)

Back Pain Explained

Many patients develop back pain following some sort of back injury. These injuries can be the result of work, play, or almost any activity performed during the activities of normal daily life. It is the normal function of the muscles surrounding the vertebrae (back bones) to immediately stiffen following any injury to the back region, even a minor sprain or strain. These muscles stiffen because it is their very important job to protect the vertebrae and your very precious spine inside.

Normally, after the injury has healed and resolved, these back muscles gradually lose their stiffness and return to their normal, relaxed state. But in some instances, for unknown reasons these muscles remain in a state of stiffness and eventually may stay in a constant state of spasm, which is called *myofascial pain syndrome*. This state of constant spasm can be compared to having a chronic charley horse in the muscles of the lower back.

If the muscles of your lower back get into this constant state of stiffness and spasm, you are a prime candidate for the Vicious Cycle of Chronic Pain (see chapter 14). With each movement of your back, these stiff muscles can go into a deeper spasm, causing you more pain, which in turn causes you to tighten these muscles more and use them less. With each episode of pain, your brain tells you, "Be careful, you are hurting yourself and causing damage," though in this case it is not true. It is therefore understandable that with time, the back pain patient moves his or her back less and less (in an effort to protect it), resulting in even more muscle stiffness, and causing the pain to spread and lead to a greater loss of muscle function. Thus, you get caught in the tangled web of the Vicious Cycle of Chronic Pain.

The actual medical problem lies within the muscle and the fascia, the bands of fibrous tissue that cover and attach muscles, ligaments, and tendons. The muscle and fascia in the lower back become and stay stiff, spastic, and tender. The actual reason why this happens is unknown. However, it is believed that the risk factors for developing myofascial pain are injury, repetitive movements, and lack of stretching and exercise of the involved muscles and fascia.

Many different theories about what's wrong in the muscle have been proposed, such as chemical abnormalities, oxygenation problems, and microscopic muscle tears, but none of these potential underlying factors have accumulated good scientific evidence to prove they are the primary biological cause for chronic spasm and pain.

The Natural Course of Back Pain

If active movement of the involved muscles does not occur, the back muscles continue to be spastic and painful. Additionally, because the back pain sufferer starts to overuse other muscles to compensate, there is often a gradual spreading of pain to other body parts, such as the hips, buttocks, and even legs, as these other muscles eventually become spastic due to overuse and abnormal use. Therefore, if not treated appropriately, the natural course of back pain can become very stressful and disabling, and even scary as you feel the pain spread. However, remember that the good news is that if properly treated, most people's back pain is potentially curable! **Yes, we did say curable!**

CONCLUSION: SEE A PAIN SPECIALIST AND TAKE PART IN AN ACTIVE PT PROGRAM

Back pain is probably the most common cause of chronic pain. Unfortunately, most doctors and even some so-called "pain specialists" are not properly trained in how to diagnose or treat this condition. As is the case with many chronic pain conditions, simply taking medication or getting nerve blocks will not resolve the problem. The most important type of treatment is an active PT program, although other types of treatment can help. It is crucial that you work with a knowledgeable physician and a physical therapist to create a treatment regimen specific to your underlying problem. With the right mix of therapies and especially an active PT program, back pain is actually curable.

(Get the Facts: continued)

Fact 3: Back surgery may make no difference in your long-term prognosis. Several studies have found that one year after having surgery for low back pain, there is absolutely no difference in the amount of pain between those who had back surgery and those who did not, even with the same degree of disc bulge.

Fact 4: If you have back pain, don't see a surgeon in an area where there are lots of back surgeons! Studies have shown that the number of back surgeries performed in any given geographic area in the United States does not correlate with the number of people who live in that area or with the number of hard labor-type jobs, but rather with the number of doctors in that area who perform back surgery for a living. You know that old saying: "If all you have is a hammer, everything looks like a nail." In other words, because orthopedic surgeons and neurosurgeons are trained (and get paid) to do surgery, they are more likely to perform surgery on people in pain. You don't need to move away from these areas; just make sure you don't see only a surgeon who treats pain only by cutting.

29

Q & A *with*
Dr. Argoff and Dr. Galer

What do you typically recommend for your patients with back pain?

Luckily, we've worked in multidisciplinary pain centers with a team of experts including physical therapists, pain psychologists, and others. Most often, we prescribe a topical drug or an oral NSAID or COX-2 drug. And we always have our back pain patients begin an active PT program. We also most often have each patient assessed by a pain psychologist and treated for any psychological condition he or she may have due to the back pain.

Why do so many people with back pain get nerve blocks or surgery?

Hmmm. It's hard to be diplomatic about this, so to put it bluntly:

• Most doctors are not appropriately trained to evaluate back pain.

• Too many "back specialists" make their income from performing procedures such as nerve blocks and spinal cord stimulation, or at least make a lot more money doing these things.

• Insurance companies will pay for five nerve blocks and two surgeries more readily than other types of treatments that are likely to be more effective and carry less risk.

• Patients want a quick and simple cure.

CHAPTER 2

Getting a Grip on Neck Pain

Trigger point injections

can offer lasting relief.

Neck Pain:
A Patient's Story

I've always had some minor neck pain that comes and goes—nothing major, just sort of a "crick" in my neck, especially when I spent a lot of time on the computer for a few days straight. However, about six months ago, I was involved in a fender-bender and the pain in my neck has been constant. It feels like deep aching in my neck, and over the past few months, I've also been getting bad headaches and some shoulder pain.

the PRESCRIPTION *for* NECK PAIN

Treatments for neck pain aim to reduce the tight, spastic muscles in the neck and, often, the shoulders.

The optimal prescription is multimodal therapy, where the most critical treatment is an active physical therapy (PT) program. Medication can reduce the pain to make the PT program more productive. In addition, "nontraditional" treatments such as acupuncture can help. Also, many of the psychological treatments discussed in this book can make a big difference for many patients with neck pain.

- ✓ Medications for pain
- ✓ Active PT
- ✓ Nontraditional treatments such as acupuncture
- ✓ Psychology

Symptoms of Neck Pain

You have neck pain, most commonly described by patients as deep, aching, burning, and sharp. For most people, the pain spreads beyond their neck, so it shouldn't be surprising if your pain shoots into your shoulders and arms or is accompanied by a headache. Many patients with neck pain also complain of feeling dizzy and lightheaded. This is because the muscles in the neck actually play a role in keeping our bodies balanced (so that we don't fall) by telling our brain the location of our head. Thus, when these muscles go into spasm, they can give the brain misinformation and cause a feeling of lightheadedness.

Much like chronic back pain, there are many causes of neck pain. And like back pain, too often people are told (or self-diagnose) that their pain is due to a disc bulge, a pinched nerve in the neck, or arthritis. Most of the time this is incorrect. In fact, the most common cause of neck pain, like back pain, is prolonged tight and spastic muscles (myofascial pain), and that's what we will focus on in this chapter.

Pain Alert!

Trigger Point or Disc Bulge? Muscles, ligaments, and tendons all can be affected by myofascial dysfunction and develop tight, tender focal areas, or what you might call "tight knots." These tender regions of your muscles, ligaments, or tendons are called *trigger points*.

Trigger points cause pain not only locally, but also—or sometimes only—in areas that are distant from the trigger point (known as *referred pain*). Trigger points in certain neck muscles can cause you to have pain in your shoulder and arm and can even cause tension-type headaches. If you are a migraine sufferer, they may bring on one of these headaches.

Therefore, you and your doctor must realize that just because the pain may shoot from your neck and into your arms does not necessarily mean the pain is from a disc bulge or from a nerve root being squeezed in the neck. Many doctors assume this is the case, leading to a wrong diagnosis and inappropriate treatment, and sometimes even unwarranted neck surgery. Be careful!

Medications for Neck Pain

NSAIDS/COX-2 INHIBITORS RELIEVE PAIN

At times, some patients do find slight to moderate relief using prescription-strength nonsteroidal anti-inflammatory drugs (NSAIDs) and COX-2 inhibitor medications. These medications reduce inflammation and also can have a direct pain-relieving effect. It is very important to consider the potential serious side effects of these drugs, even if bought over the counter. If taken too often or at too high a dose, they can cause major liver, kidney, and heart problems. However, for some patients, these medications can provide good pain relief without intolerable side effects, when taken as recommended. Read the label and follow the recommended dosing.

THE LIDOCAINE PATCH 5% WORKS ON THE SPOT

Although it is not FDA-approved to treat neck pain, some patients have reported obtaining some pain relief with Lidoderm. Lidocaine, the active medicine in Lidoderm, acts directly on pain nerves in the skin and muscles to quiet down the intensity of the pain signals they are producing. Because Lidoderm is a topical drug, there are no known serious side effects and no drug interactions to worry about. The FDA-approved dosing for lidocaine patch 5% is up to three patches at a time applied to the painful area twelve hours on and then twelve hours off. However, many studies have been published showing that it is safe to use up to four patches at a time, keeping them on for twenty-four hours and then putting on new patches.

TOPICAL NSAIDS HAVE MINIMAL SERIOUS SIDE EFFECTS

Although not studied for the treatment of neck pain, topical NSAID medications are frequently used outside the United States for treating neck pain. Because these are topical drugs, there are no known serious side effects and no drug interactions to be concerned about; except very rarely all diclofenac products may cause liver abnormalities. These drugs directly infuse anti-inflammatory agents into the inflamed muscles, ligaments, and tendons. Topical NSAIDs are not FDA-approved to treat neck pain, but they are approved to treat osteoarthritis and acute minor sports injury pain. Currently FDA-approved and available topical NSAID lotions and gels are applied four times daily to the painful region; the recommendation for the Flector Patch is one patch daily, to be replaced by a new patch.

TRAMADOL WORKS IN TWO WAYS

Tramadol is an interesting drug with two different pain-relieving mechanisms in the spine and brain: one on the nervous system's opioid system and the other on the neurotransmitters norepinephrine and serotonin. Several good studies show that some patients with back pain experience significant pain relief with tramadol, without intolerable side effects. Thus, it is likely neck pain patients may obtain relief from tramadol as well.

OPIOIDS ARE CAUTIOUSLY RECOMMENDED TO CERTAIN PATIENTS

Opioid medication can benefit certain sufferers of neck pain. Like all medications for this condition, opioids are not a cure, but when prescribed appropriately for the right patient they can help a patient participate in a needed active PT program. Opioids work by directly interacting with natural opioid systems in the spinal cord and brain and also likely on the peripheral nerves. They should not be prescribed as first-line therapy because of their predilection for causing side effects and because of the rare occurrences of addiction and diversion (someone taking your pills for a high or to sell for money). However, for patients who are severely debilitated from their neck pain and for whom nothing else has worked, opioids can be a godsend.

Neck Alert!

Be "Smart Active" When Your Pain Isn't Bad When you find a medication that relieves your neck pain, it is crucial that you use the pain-free periods to take part in the PT treatments that will get to the core of the problem.

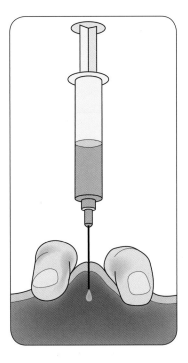

▲ Trigger Point Injection

Nonmedication Therapies for Neck Pain

Following are the most important therapies in treating neck pain caused by myofascial problems, the most common cause of neck pain. One or more of these are absolutely necessary to get to the root and truly resolve the problem causing the pain.

ACTIVE PT IS NUMBER ONE

An active PT program is by far the most important treatment for patients with neck pain. The most important goal of this treatment is for the patient to gradually increase the use of the involved neck muscles with stretching, strengthening, and endurance exercises.

When initiating a PT program, expect the pain to get slightly worse during the first few sessions. It is important to realize that this worsening is a good sign, as it means the muscles responsible for your chronic pain are the ones receiving the needed treatment.

ACUPUNCTURE CAN PROVIDE SIGNIFICANT RELIEF

Many neck pain patients obtain significant pain relief with a series of acupuncture treatments performed by a trained acupuncturist. Though studies lack substantial evidence, we recommend acupuncture as a safe and potentially helpful treatment for neck pain because we've seen very good results in some patients. No one truly knows how acupuncture works, but Chinese medicine claims it manipulates underlying energies, a theory unrelated to our Western medicine's anatomical and physiological tenets and beliefs.

TRIGGER POINT INJECTIONS (TPIs) FIND THE TROUBLE SPOT

TPIs are just what the name implies—injections aimed directly into the tight, spastic region of the muscle. Depending on doctor preference, TPIs can be done by using an acupuncture needle (also called dry-needling), or by injecting a local anesthetic such as lidocaine, a steroid, or both a local anesthetic and a steroid. In our experience for some patients, dry-needling may be the best method as it seems to work as well as the others, but without injecting a drug into the body. Other patients report that injection of lidocaine and/or a steroid works better for them.

Evidence suggests that TPIs can relieve neck pain for days, weeks, or months in some patients. However, all patients should be warned that the initial few injections can be quite painful. The muscle may actually go into a deeper spasm before it eventually relaxes. Patients usually notice a dramatic increase in their ability to move their neck and shoulders after TPIs. The key with TPIs is for the patient to

▼ HOW BOTOX WORKS

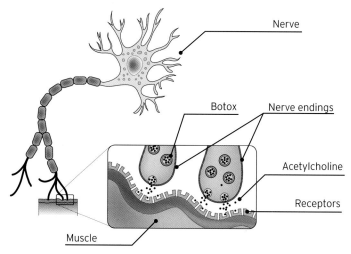

What's New: Botox for Pain?

Over the past several years, some pain doctors have been injecting botulinum toxin (Botox, Myobloc, Dysport) into trigger points.

How does that work to relieve pain? This toxin (yes, the same one used by Hollywood types to remove wrinkles!) works by blocking a muscle chemical, acetylcholine, which keeps the muscle unable to contract or go into spasm for several months. Other chemicals that may cause pain, inlcuding Substance P, glutamate, and CGRP, may also be blocked by a certain type of this toxin. Although this treatment appears to work for some patients with a longer duration of muscle trigger-point relaxation, it's not clear whether it provides advantages over the older TPI techniques for all patients. It may be that just inserting a needle into the myofascial trigger point (dry-needling) may be equally effective for many patients.

simultaneously undergo active PT to retrain the muscle to stay in a relaxed state.

Most pain doctors recommend an initial trial of weekly TPIs for four to six weeks, and then reassessment to see if the patient is experiencing a positive outcome. Again, remember it is of utmost importance that during this TPI trial, the patient is also enrolled in an active PT program.

HEAT TREATMENT PROVIDES TEMPORARY RELIEF

With the advent of a new type of heat wrap (ThermaCare), we have seen many advertisements touting the use of this type of therapy for all types of pain, including neck pain. Although there is not a great deal of evidence to support heat wrap therapy in the treatment of neck pain, it may provide some temporary relief for some neck pain patients without causing any side effects or risks.

CRANIOSACRAL THERAPY HAS NO SIDE EFFECTS

Some patients with neck pain obtain significant pain relief and improved function with craniosacral release therapy and osteopathic manipulation performed by trained therapists. Though we as neurologists do not understand or believe in the theory of underlying biowaves and cerebrospinal waves that are at the core of craniosacral therapy, we have to admit we've had several patients with neck pain report tremendous benefit from craniosacral release treatments. And there are no side effects.

What's New: Do-It-Yourself Hot Trigger Point Release

One emerging type of heat treatment uses a focused heat source aimed directly at the myofascial trigger point. Called *focal heat trigger-point (FHTP) therapy*, this novel treatment acts just like a TPI, but you can do it yourself instead of having to go to a doctor's office for treatment. We've had some success in treating patients with FHTP, although at the time of this writing no studies had been conducted.

Can I buy a device for this at the drugstore? As of the writing of this book, no device is specifically marketed as an FHTP treatment. However, one device, called Zeno, is available in some drugstores and online. FDA-approved to treat acne, this device has a focused heat source and a timer that regulates the amount of heat applied to the skin so as not to cause a burn.

How do I know where to point the device? It's simple. Find the tight, tender knots in your muscles, ligaments, and tendons (see "Examination Findings: Trigger Points in the Neck") and apply the focal heat source with a moderate degree of pressure on the skin overlying the trigger point.

THERAPEUTIC MASSAGE AND ACUPRESSURE WORK FOR SOME

Some evidence suggests that therapeutic massage and acupressure therapy may benefit some patients with neck pain. As with other therapies, such treatments should be paired with an active PT/exercise program.

STRESS MANAGEMENT TECHNIQUES RELAX THE MUSCLES

The stress reaction (as fully described in chapter 17) has been shown to cause a worsening of muscle spasms in muscles that are causing neck pain. Therefore, it makes sense that stress management techniques, such as relaxation, imagery, and biofeedback (see chapter 11), can play a very important role in the treatment of neck pain.

PSYCHOLOGICAL TREATMENTS RELIEVE THE MIND AND NECK

Many neck pain patients have depression from the constant, debilitating pain they experience. Also, many patients whose pain began after an accident such as a whiplash injury may have post-traumatic stress disorder. If you have any of these psychological conditions, you should seek psychological treatment, as this therapy will help to relieve not only your psychological problem, but also your pain (see chapter 11 for more about depression and anxiety).

Therapies to Avoid in Managing Neck Pain
PASSIVE PT WILL NOT WORK

Unfortunately, many PT programs focus on passive, "touchy-feely" therapies, such as gentle massage, ultrasound, and warm baths. Although these types of PT techniques may make you feel better temporarily, they will not treat, resolve, or cure your neck problem.

NERVE BLOCKS ARE NOT THE ANSWER

Most pain medicine authorities agree that there is no role for nerve blocks in the treatment of chronic neck pain for the majority of patients.

SPINAL CORD STIMULATION IS A VERY LAST RESORT

Although there is evidence that spinal cord stimulation may be of benefit to some patients with various types of neck pain, it is our opinion that this should be reserved as a very last resort for patients with neck pain.

SURGERY IS NOT USUALLY THE FIX FOR NECK PAIN

Many patients are incorrectly told by their doctors and surgeons that their neck pain is caused by a surgically correctable problem, when in reality the problem is due to chronic myofascial dysfunction. There is absolutely no role for surgery in the treatment of neck pain associated with myofascial pain, the most common cause of neck pain. However, there are uncommon medical conditions that cause neck pain where surgery may be warranted, as we describe in "Less Common Causes of Neck Pain" later in this chapter.

MUSCLE RELAXANTS ARE REALLY SEDATIVES

Although drug companies have for years marketed the following drugs as "muscle relaxants," in reality they do not have any true muscle relaxant properties! No drug has been shown to significantly undo the spasm of chronic myofascial conditions. Because these drugs act more like Valium, causing significant sedation, we don't recommend them for most patients.

Carisoprodol (Soma)
Baclofen (Lioresal)
Cyclobenzaprine (Flexeril)
Dantrolene (Dantrium)
Metaxalone (Skelaxin)
Methocarbamol (Robaxin)
Orphenadrine (Norflex)

Diagnosing Neck Pain

Radiology tests, such as X-rays, CT scans, and magnetic resonance imaging (MRI), are often normal (though remember that many middle-age and older persons have bulging discs in their necks that are not responsible for their neck pain). Electromyography (EMG) may or may not demonstrate abnormal muscle spasms. The results of an EMG are most often completely normal in people with neck pain.

Examination Findings: Trigger Points in the Neck

The neurological examination in patients with neck pain due to myofascial dysfunction is completely normal. However, definite abnormalities are found on direct examination of the muscles of the neck. When the doctor assesses the neck muscles, he or she will find myofascial trigger points, tight and tender muscles that are painful. Quite often, gently pushing on trigger points will reproduce all of the pains that a neck pain patient experiences.

Less Common Causes Of Neck Pain

The vast majority of neck pain is due to myofascial dysfunction in the muscles of the neck and shoulders. However, there are less common causes of neck pain that you should be aware of. We described several of these in chapter 1 on back pain, such as spinal stenosis and ankylosing spondylitis, although here the problem is in the neck region. Some other less common causes of neck pain include the following:

CERVICAL SPONDOLYTIC MYELOPATHY
What is it?
This condition is probably the most common cause of spinal cord problems in adults older than fifty-five. With age, degenerative changes occur in many components of the cervical (neck) spine, including in the vertebral joints, the intervertebral discs, and the ligaments and connective tissue. With these changes, eventually the spinal cord becomes squeezed.

Diagnosis:
On neurological examination:
- The patient complains of abnormal weakness and sensory perception in the arms. In severe cases, the legs may function abnormally as the condition progresses.
- Muscle wasting (loss of muscle bulk) may be evident in the hand and fingers.
- Abnormal reflexes
- Upon flexing of the neck, the patient may feel an electrical sensation down the back (Lhermitte's sign).
- An MRI or CT scan shows abnormal narrowing of the cervical spinal canal.

Symptoms:
- The patient has a stiff neck.
- Crepitus (grating, creeks, and pops) are felt and heard in the neck with movement.
- Weakness; sharp, shooting pains; dull, achy sensations; and numbness or tingling in the arms and hands are common.
- With chronic severe disease, weakness in the legs and feet and stiffness and imbalance with walking occur.

Treatment:
- This is one of the rare cases where many experts recommend early surgical treatment to open the cervical canal space.

OSTEOPOROSIS
What is it?
Osteoporosis is a chronic condition where the bones become weak and brittle due to loss of bone density. This is very common, with at least 20 percent of women over the age of 50 having osteoporosis. All bones become weak and can fracture. When the neck bone (cervical vertebrae) fractures, it can cause chronic neck pain.

Neck Pain Explained

Many patients develop neck pain following an accident that resulted in a whiplash type of injury. When an accident involves your neck, it is the normal function of the muscles surrounding your vertebrae (i.e., neck bones) to immediately stiffen to protect your vertebrae and your precious cervical spinal cord which is guarded by your vertebrae. Usually after a few days or weeks, these muscles gradually lose their stiffness and return to their normal relaxed tone. However, for unknown reasons, in some people these muscles remain in a stiff and spastic state, eventually settling into a constant state of spasm, like a chronic charley horse in your neck muscles.

Sometimes people who work at a computer all day can develop neck pain because they are overusing their neck muscles. Your body and neck weren't made to be held still, staring at a computer screen for hours and hours. So, again, make sure to stretch, and if you're feeling sore, take a break and don't overuse those muscles.

The Natural Course of Neck Pain

If you get into the Vicious Cycle of Chronic Pain (see chapter 14) with your neck pain, the news isn't good. But if you start a program that is focused on gradually moving the muscles of your neck to relax them and get them moving on a regular basis, the news is great: You can completely resolve your neck pain! So, if you're afraid of moving your neck for fear of causing pain and fear of potentially causing a spine problem, you're actually causing more problems—more neck spasms, more neck stiffness, and a spreading of your pain. The future is in your hands (and neck).

CONCLUSION: NECK PAIN IS COMMON AND TREATABLE

Neck pain is a widespread problem and is curable for the vast majority of sufferers. However, many treatment options are available for most patients. If you are suffering from this condition, you should speak with your doctor about these options to alleviate your pain so that you can function at your full potential. Certainly, more than 99 percent of you do not need surgery and can be cured of your pain problem with the therapies we have discussed.

Neck Alert!

Before You See a Chiropractor... Studies have shown that chiropractic manipulations can help some patients with neck pain. However, it is of the utmost importance that you make sure you do not have any neurological abnormalities in your neck prior to receiving chiropractic manipulation. Such abnormalities may be experienced as weakness, numbness, or tingling in your hands or fingers. However, you may not have any symptoms, and your spine abnormality would be diagnosed only on neurological examination, manifested by abnormal reflexes or sensory and motor abnormalities (that you may not notice yourself).

The spinal cord is one of your most vital organs and is quite vulnerable in the neck. It is known that certain chiropractic manipulations of the neck can cause very serious and permanent damage (paralysis) if performed on patients with neurological neck disease. Therefore, before you see a chiropractor for your neck pain, you should have a neurological examination from a neurologist to ensure that you do not have any signs of potential neck neurological abnormalities.

How do I avoid developing neck pain associated with my occupation?

Remember, you have neck muscles that need to move on a regular basis. In this day and age of computers, we all need to remember to stretch our necks every ten to twenty minutes.

My doctor thinks I need surgery in my neck for pain, now that I have pain that radiates from my neck into my fingers. He says I must have a pinched nerve. But you are telling me I likely do not need surgery. What should I do?

We've put you in a tough spot, but maybe we've saved you from unnecessary and risky surgery. We recommend that you seek an evaluation from a neurologist with pain medicine training, hopefully one who works in a pain center and is experienced in diagnosing myofascial pain. We also recommend that you ask the doctor recommending neck surgery if he has evaluated you for myofascial neck dysfunction. If he hasn't, definitely do not jump into surgery with this doctor.

CHAPTER 3

Conquering Arthritis
(OA/RA)

Breakthrough drugs significantly reduce pain and disability.

The Pain and Disability of Arthritis

There are hundreds of types of arthritis, and all have one thing in common: One or more joints in the body become inflamed and dysfunctional, usually resulting in pain and disability. Overall, approximately 43 million people in the United States currently have some form of arthritis including the types discussed here, and in 2020 that number is projected to increase to about sixty million. So, as you can see, arthritis is very common and is only going to become more prevalent. It is very likely that every American by the year 2020 will either have some type of arthritis or know of a family member, friend, or colleague who is suffering from an inflamed joint disorder.

The two most common types of arthritis are osteoarthritis (OA) and rheumatoid arthritis (RA). OA affects almost 30 million people in the United States, and RA afflicts 2 million; both cause significant pain and disability. Worldwide, it has been estimated that a whopping 10 percent of adults sixty years or older have OA, and almost 1 percent of the world's population suffers from RA. The pain, disability, and suffering caused by these two conditions are enormous in every corner of our world.

BREAKTHROUGHS IN TREATMENT OFFER HOPE

Luckily for OA and RA sufferers, there have been significant breakthroughs in treatment in the past decade. Science has begun to unravel the underlying causes of these conditions and the pain associated with them, resulting in much-improved treatments. Two such breakthroughs are the disease-modifying antirheumatic drugs (DMARDs) and new topical nonsteroidal anti-inflammatory drugs (NSAIDs), which we will discuss later in this chapter. And with the significant amount of funding and effort put into studying arthritis throughout the world, both in academic centers and in the pharmaceutical industry, it seems like every month new insights are gained in OA and RA that may eventually have a direct impact on further improving the lives of people living with these conditions.

In this chapter, we will focus on these two common forms of arthritis, discussing OA first and then RA. If you are not sure what type of arthritis you (or your family member, friend, or colleague) may have, you are not alone, since they share many similarities. Please refer to the table below, which describes their differences. But as always, we suggest that you be evaluated and examined by a trained physician, one who specializes in all types of arthritis: a *rheumatologist*.

▼ TABLE 3.1

Symptom	OA	RA
Age of onset	< 45 for men, > 55 for women	Any age
Joints affected	Usually the weight-bearing joints, such as knees and hips, as well as the small finger joint closest to the fingernail Most often starts on one side of the body, and not all these joints are initially affected	Most commonly on both sides of the body at the same time
Joint symptoms	Pain Usually only mild swelling Morning stiffness usually felt < 1 hour	Pain Moderate to severe swelling Morning stiffness felt > 1 hour
Speed of onset	Very slow over many years	Varies; may be very slow over many years or rapidly from weeks to months
Nonjoint symptoms	Not present	Frequent, including fatigue, generally feeling ill, fever, weight loss
Involvement of other body parts/organs	No	May involve lung, eye, nerves, and blood vessels
Gender	Affects women and men equally	Affects women more than men

The Onset of OA:
A Patient's Story

It started out in one of my knees. In my early fifties, I began to notice that when I was walking in the mall, my left knee started to ache after walking for about thirty minutes. I thought it was just due to getting old and gaining some weight, but then when my other knee began to have pain and Tylenol stopped working, I saw my doctor, who told me it was osteoarthritis. Now that I'm almost sixty-five, I've also noticed that whenever I paint (my hobby is oil painting), my finger joints will ache after several hours of painting, which had never happened before. It's bearable; lots of friends have other things worse than arthritis, but I gotta tell you, pretty soon it's going to be difficult for me to paint and play with my grandchildren.

the PRESCRIPTION *for* OSTEOARTHRITIS

A self-help program is the first line of treatment for OA patients: exercise, healthy eating habits, and losing weight if obese.

Medications can often provide enough relief with minimal side effects for patients to maintain their exercise and physical therapy (PT). For severe and debilitating cases of OA, injections may be used to restore fluid, and as a last resort, surgery (including knee and hip replacement) is usually successful.

- ✓ Exercising and eating right
- ✓ Medications for pain relief and injections for pain relief
- ✓ Nonmedication treatments
- ✓ Surgery

The Symptoms of OA

You have OA pain: deep, sharp, or aching pain in your fingers, feet, knees, or hips. OA may also affect the neck and back (spinal vertebrae). It typically first affects the joints that are used often and bear the brunt of your weight, such as your knees and hips. The pain of OA is always in the involved joint, which also may be tender to the touch. Many patients say the pain gets worse later in the day. Patients with chronic, severe OA may have near-constant pain in their OA joints.

An OA joint may have some swelling, warmth, and a feeling of creaking. Most patients with OA also complain of joint stiffness, especially in the morning. In some patients with an aggressive, progressive type of OA, the joints may become deformed. As with most other chronic pain conditions, patients with OA will have different types and degrees of symptoms.

▼ **NORMAL JOINT (LEFT) VERSUS JOINT WITH OSTEOARTHRITIS (RIGHT)**

Muscle
Bursa
Bone
Synovial membrane
Synovial fluid
Joint capsule
Cartilage
Thinned cartilage
Bone ends rub together

Who Gets OA?

Men and women are equally afflicted with OA. However, males more often get OA before age forty-five, whereas after age fifty-five it occurs more frequently in females. Although all races can develop OA, there appears to be a higher likelihood in Japanese people and lower incidences in South African black, East Indian, and Chinese people.

Following are the risk factors for OA, independent of age and race:

Genetic: Some people inherit a defective gene that appears to make abnormal cartilage, making them prone to OA.

Joint injury: An injury to a joint, such as a knee, predisposes a person to developing OA later in life in that joint.

Obesity: Putting more weight on the knee and hip joints increases the risk of those joints developing OA. This is something you can control!

47

OA Treatment, Step by Step

The treatment plan for OA starts from the simplest things you can do to help your-self with the most benign treatments and least risky drugs, such as over-the-counter (OTC) medication or topical NSAIDs, to more invasive and riskier treatments, such as an injection or surgery.

Medications To Treat OA Pain

Though different types of medication have been found to relieve OA pain, it is important to remember that medication is only part of the treatment equation. Medication should be used to assist the daily routine of exercise of an OA joint. All medications described in this section require a doctor's prescription, except for some of the classic NSAIDs (Motrin, Advil, and Aleve) as well as acetaminophen (Tylenol).

NSAIDS AND COX-2 INHIBITORS REDUCE INFLAMMATION

For most patients and doctors, these drugs, taken orally, are the mainstay of treatment for OA pain and disability. NSAIDs such as aspirin and ibuprofen work by blocking the enzyme cyclooxygenase, or COX, that is involved in causing inflammation. COX has two forms: COX-1 and COX-2. COX-1 protects the stomach lining from acids and other digestive chemicals and helps maintain normal kidney function. COX-2 is produced when joints are injured or inflamed. Traditional NSAIDs block the actions of both COX-1 and COX-2, which is why they can cause stomach upset and bleeding as well as ease pain and inflammation. COX-2 inhibitors such as Celebrex selectively work only on COX-2, and thereby were thought to be safer than traditional NSAIDS but were shown to have other adverse effects; more on this shortly. These types of drugs reduce pain by affecting joint inflammation and, when taken orally, may also have direct pain-relieving actions in the spinal cord.

ACETAMINOPHEN RELIEVES PAIN WITH FEW SIDE EFFECTS

Acetaminophen (Tylenol) is one of the most commonly used medications to treat the pain of OA. Studies have shown that this OTC drug gives many patients good pain alleviation without side effects. However, use this drug with caution; acetaminophen overuse is the number one cause of liver damage and liver transplants in the United States!

LIDOCAINE PATCH 5% (LIDODERM) DULLS THE PAIN SIGNAL

Although not FDA-approved to treat OA pain, lidocaine has been shown in several studies to provide good pain relief and no serious side effects when delivered by a patch around an OA joint. Lidocaine Patch was FDA approved in 1999 for the treatment of a chronic nerve injury pain called *postherpetic neuralgia*, and it is available by prescription. Interestingly, many doctors and pain scientists were surprised when Lidoderm helped to relieve OA pain. Now, we realize that in OA (and other forms of arthritis), the pain nerves in the joint become sensitive to inflammation; the lidocaine from the lidocaine patch diffuses into the joint to decrease the pain signals coming from these joint pain nerves.

TRAMADOL WORKS IN THE CENTRAL NERVOUS SYSTEM

Tramadol has been shown in multiple studies to relieve OA pain. Tramadol works on two different pain pathways in the brain and spinal cord: those that use natural opioids and those that use the neurochemical norepinephrine and serotonin. By working on these pathways in the central nervous system, tramadol may diminish the amount of pain being felt.

DULOXETINE (CYMBALTA) IS GOOD FOR KNEE OA

Recently, several good scientific studies have demonstrated that duloxetine relieves the pain of knee OA. Duloxetine works on neurochemicals in the brain and spinal cord that are involved in both pain and depression, norepinephrine and serotonin. However, like many antidepressants that work for pain, duloxetine alleviates pain even if the patient is not depressed, without any effects on mood, wakefulness, or thinking abilities.

OPIOIDS (NARCOTICS) FOR HARD-TO-TREAT CASES

Over the past decade, many different opioid medications have been shown in clinical trials to reduce moderate to severe OA pain in patients who have not responded adequately to acetaminophen and NSAIDs/COX-2 drugs. These prescription drugs are most commonly prescribed in pill or capsule (but also in patch) form, and they work in the pain processing regions of the brain and spinal cord, where natural opioid-like neurochemicals exist, to naturally help reduce pain sensations. In addition, these drugs may also have an effect locally. In our opinion, as with other chronic pain conditions, opioids should not be prescribed as first-line medications, but should be prescribed for hard-to-treat OA patients with moderate to severe refractory pain that fails to respond to other medication types. Those pa-

OA Alert!

Take NSAIDs with Care
When taken in recommended doses, NSAIDs and COX-2 inhibitors can be very helpful. However, if consumed too frequently or at too high a dose, they can cause potentially serious side effects, even when the OTC NSAIDs Motrin, Advil, and Aleve are used. Incorrect use may lead to serious liver, kidney, and heart problems. If one of these types of medications doesn't provide you with meaningful relief or gives you intolerable side effects, try a few others to find one that provides relief without the side effects.

What's New: OA

Topical NSAIDs Gain FDA Approval Topical drugs are applied to the skin overlying the painful OA joint and then penetrate the skin to work directly in the joint. The drug is directly delivered to where it is needed, with very little getting into the bloodstream and none of it getting into your stomach, producing many fewer side effects than if you took the drug in pill or capsule form by mouth.

What kinds of OA do they treat? Pennsaid has been shown in multiple studies to not only treat the pain of knee OA, but also improve function and overall health in OA patients. Voltaren Gel has been shown to improve the pain of knee and hand OA. Also, several studies have shown Pennsaid to be as effective as an oral NSAID in treating the signs and symptoms of OA, with a reduction in some of the side effects. Both Pennsaid and Voltaren Gel are applied to the skin overlying the OA joint four-times-per-day. Also available is a topical NSAID patch, Flector, which is FDA-approved

(continued)

tients should be monitored to see if the opioids significantly reduce pain without intolerable side effects such as feeling overly sedated and having trouble thinking. If you experience bad side effects or poor pain relief with one opioid, you may want to try another, since many patients respond poorly to one and well with to another. Be aware of the risk of addiction and the potential for misuse and diversion (someone taking your pills for a high or to sell for money) that accompanies these types of medications.

HYALURONIC ACID JOINT INJECTIONS REPLACE NATURAL LUBRICANT

In our joints, a natural viscous liquid called *hyaluronan* acts as a lubricator, helping the joints move smoothly and absorb shocks. With OA, hyaluronan becomes thinner, making it less effective. The concept of hyaluronic acid joint injections is to replace some of the thinning hyaluronan with a thicker, better-working liquid. The typical course of therapy is one injection per week for three to five weeks.

The FDA has approved several formulations of hyaluronic acid for injection into the knee, and some doctors have injected this into other OA joints as well without good studies to support such use. These injections are recommended only after regular exercise and medication have failed to relieve the pain and symptoms of OA.

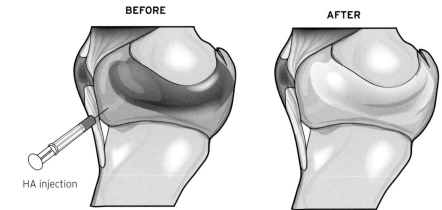

BEFORE   AFTER

HA injection

▲ Hyaluronic acid joint injections

SURGERY AS A LAST RESORT

When the pain and disability of knee or hip OA become severe and all other therapies have failed, a total knee or hip replacement can be life-changing for patients.
Although it sounds like a drastic procedure, knee and hip replacement surgery has
become commonplace and safe, revolutionizing the treatment of severe OA. So,
unlike most other surgeries performed to relieve pain, total knee or hip replacement is highly recommended for folks with debilitating OA pain that has not responded to other treatments. We have seen our patients and family members alike
get a new lease on life with new joints thanks to such surgeries.

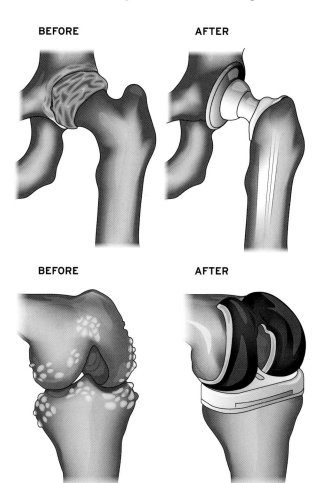

▲ Hip (above) and Knee (below) replacements

(What's New: OA continued)

to treat acute pain associated with
sports injuries, such as sprains and
strains. The problem with Flector
is that it hasn't been studied in
placebo controlled studies of OA
and also many patients complain
that it doesn't stay in place,
especially when applied over joints.

**How are Topical NSAIDs differ-
ent from OTC topical ointments?**
Topical NSAIDs have an active
medication, and therefore require
a prescription. The commonly
used OTC topical remedies such
as Bengay, Aspercreme, Icy Hot,
SALONPAS, and Zostrix did not require any studies for FDA approval
since they do not have a real drug
within them or because the FDA
"grandfathered" their approval
without the need to prove effectiveness. They are all considered
counterirritants, having chemicals,
such as menthol, salicylates, or
low-dose capsaicin, that cause irritation of the skin and result in a
feeling of warmth or cooling, with
the idea that the warm or cooling
sensation helps to cover up the
pain of OA. Recent scientific re-
views of studies that evaluated all
of the counterirritants for OA pain
have concluded that these OTC
remedies do not have any meaningful effect on OA pain.

Nonmedication Treatments for OA

Nonmedication treatments—in particular, exercise and physical or occupational therapy—are the most important elements of treating OA, the point being to maintain joint mobility and function. Although pain relief is important, regular exercise and use of the OA joint can help to slow the deterioration of the joint.

EXERCISE AND PT ARE CORE TO THE PROGRAM

Active exercise—whether at home, in a gym, or in a PT program—is the most important type of treatment for OA. This recommendation is for all OA patients, regardless of age, the severity of the OA, or which joint is involved. The key is to use the involved joints regularly so as to maintain your ability to use them. Find an activity that you enjoy doing, such as walking, jogging, biking, or swimming; remember to do your stretching and isometric exercises; and "just do it"! You don't have to be assessed and treated by a trained physical or occupational therapist, but your overall exercise program should involve the following elements:

Stretching/range of motion of your joints:
- Do passive stretching (meaning you gently stretch the muscles, tendons, and ligaments around your joints) daily, starting with five to seven repetitions and increasing to ten repetitions per day. If possible, try to do these stretches several times per day. It is important that you stretch in a slow, steady manner, without bouncing and without stretching to the point of pain, and that you breathe regularly.

Strengthening exercises:
- No, you don't have to become Mr. or Mrs. Bodybuilder, but strengthening the muscles around your joints can decrease future damage of your joints and greatly improve your function.
- Strength training can occur as an isometric exercise in which the muscles contract without changing in length so that the joint does not move, or as an isotonic exercise in which the muscles contract and move the joint.
- Isometric exercises are recommended, especially when painful joints limit your movement. The joint and muscles do not move, but are worked against an immovable force or are held in the same position while being opposed by resistance.

You should contract the muscle being exercised with maximum force and hold it for three to six seconds; start with two to three repetitions and slowly increase to ten repetitions. Do these exercises three times per week.

Aerobic exercise should also be done three times per week:
- Find a low-impact activity that reduces the amount of weight you put on your OA joints (e.g., swimming, biking, or rowing).
- It really doesn't matter what form of exercise you do—walking, jogging, riding a bike, swimming, yoga, and so on—as long as you do it regularly and move your OA joints.
- Avoid exercises that put too much stress on your OA joints; if you have knee or hip OA, avoid climbing stairs and jogging.
- Find shoes and insoles that provide good shock absorption.

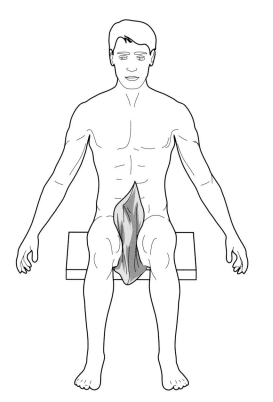
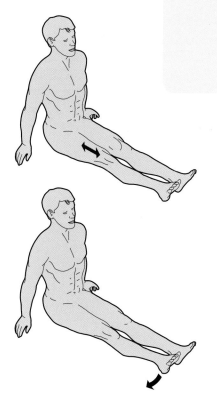

▲ Isometric exercises for the knees and hips

OA Alert!

Exercise Will Not Ruin Your Joint! Despite what old folklore and fears may tell you, active PT and exercise using your OA joint is very good for your joint, not dangerous. Many OA patients fear that because it hurts to move an OA-afflicted joint, they are causing more damage by exercising. This is not true. Experts now believe the reverse is true: Exercise will improve the function and help slow the damage of your OA joint.

53

What Are Nutraceuticals?

Nutraceuticals, sometimes called *nutritional supplements*, are extracts from certain foods that claim to have medicinal properties; the word actually comes from combining *nutrition* with *pharmaceutical*. Nutraceuticals can be taken as pills or capsules, or in a powder form in a prescribed dose, or just eaten in foods, such as the recently introduced and heavily marketed probiotic yogurts.

TRY ACUPUNCTURE WITH EXERCISE

Scientific evidence proves that acupuncture may benefit some OA patients. Although acupuncture does not replace exercise, if it provides you with some relief of your pain and symptoms, you should use it in addition to exercise.

There are many different types of acupuncture. Some acupuncturists twist the acupuncture needle as it pierces the skin, while others apply a mild electrical current to the needle. Also, sometimes an acupuncturist may apply a heated herb (moxa) to the acupuncture point instead of inserting a needle. Though ancient and used for centuries in parts of the world, it is not clear how acupuncture works. Eastern medicine practitioners believe acupuncture restores the body's energies ("yin and yang") back to a normal state.

SUPPLEMENTS/NUTRACEUTICALS IMPROVE SYMPTOMS

The most common supplement/nutraceutical recommended for OA is glucosamine combined with chondroitin sulfate. Several studies have shown that this combination nutraceutical can improve symptoms in some patients with OA. It is believed that taking glucosamine and chondroitin sulfate on a regular basis may help to restore and maintain healthy cartilage in an OA joint. Based on the fact that these nutraceuticals are safe and have been shown in some studies to benefit patients, we recommend a trial of two to three months to see if you notice any improvement. The dosages that seems to work in several studies are: glucosamine sulfate 500 milligrams taken by mouth as tablets or capsules three times daily, or once daily dosing as 1.5 grams (1,500 milligrams), and chondroitin 1200 mg per day, or 400 mg three times per day.

Another commonly used supplement comes from fish oil: omega-3. Scientific evidence suggests that this chemical can reduce inflammation, but its actual results in OA patients are not known yet. Because omega-3 can also have some other added benefits, such as improving cardiovascular health, and because there are no bad effects, we also recommend this nutraceutical.

WEIGHT LOSS DECREASES STRESS ON JOINTS

If you are overweight, losing some of that weight will reduce your OA symptoms. Losing weight will immediately decrease the stress on your OA joints and give them longer life (and give you longer life as well!). Losing weight is probably one of the most important things you can do to improve your OA pain and your overall health (in addition to quitting smoking).

Here are some simple facts based on lots of studies to further motivate you to lose weight:

- There is a strong correlation between how much pain you have with your knee and hip OA and how overweight you are.
- Being ten pounds overweight increases the force on your knees by thirty to sixty pounds with each step!
- While walking normally, a force of three to six times your body weight is put on your knees.

Compared to their healthy-weight counterparts, overweight women have four times the risk and overweight men have five times the risk of developing knee OA.

Diagnosing Osteoarthritis

There are no laboratory findings or blood tests a doctor can use to diagnose OA in a joint. However, there are certain characteristics in how the condition develops with symptoms that can help a doctor make the diagnosis. For instance, in OA of the knee, most symptoms begin after age fifty, and patients complain of morning stiffness, a grating sensation when moving the knee, and tenderness of the knee. For OA of the hand, most patients develop at least two of ten joints with bony enlargement and some deformity.

Examination Findings: OA

Very often, no definitive changes are seen on examination of an OA patient. However, in severe OA, the joint may be deformed.

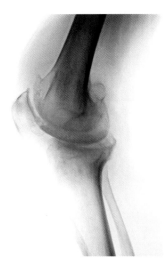

▲ X-ray of a joint with severe
Osteoarthritis

X-RAY TEST FOR OA

A regular X-ray of the joint may be very helpful in the diagnosis of OA. Typically, the X-ray will show a loss of cartilage, narrowing of the joint space, and perhaps some abnormal bone spurs. Very importantly, there is no correlation between the amount of damage in the joint seen on an X-ray and the amount of pain a patient experiences (like back pain!).

OA Pain Explained

It used to be thought that OA is caused by the natural aging process, but now most experts do not believe this is true because not every elderly person develops OA. OA is a disease of the joint—in particular, the cartilage—although all tissues in the joint may be involved, including bone, synovial, and muscle tissues. With daily use of joints over time or with injury, the cartilage begins to degenerate by flaking or forming tiny crevasses. Repetitive use of the worn joints over many years can eventually irritate and inflame the cartilage. With the gradual loss of cartilage, friction develops between the bones, causing pain and limiting joint movement. Also, cartilage inflammation can stimulate abnormal new bone outgrowths (spurs, also called *osteophytes*) around the affected joints.

Recent data seems to point to OA as being caused by an abnormal repair process in the joint, not necessarily the normal "wear and tear" of the joint. This abnormal process is what results in the loss of cartilage, inflammation of the involved joint, and sometimes, abnormal bone growth. The amount and rate of this damage vary from person to person.

The Natural Course of OA

As the symptoms of OA vary from person to person, so too does its progression. Some people have only minor involvement in one or two joints, while others find all of their joints have OA over time. However, you have some control over what happens to you! You can lose weight and exercise regularly to improve your symptoms and slow the progression of your OA.

CONCLUSION: TAKE HEART AND EXERCISE!

OA is the most common form of arthritis in the United States and often results in pain and disability of a joint, commonly in the hands, knees, and hips. Experts worldwide now recommend exercise as the number-one treatment for everyone. Luckily, lots of medications have been shown to be effective in safely treating OA pain. Lastly, if you are an OA sufferer and you are overweight, you can do yourself a huge favor by losing some weight.

My mother had OA in her hand, and so did my grandmother. Now I am seeing some symptoms of OA too. Am I helpless in what I can do?

Definitely not! You can take control of your OA by exercising regularly, using all of your joints, including your hands (see Exercise and PT Maintain Mobility, p. 64, describing hand exercises); losing weight if you are overweight (being overweight does affect the hands!); taking the supplements glucosamine and chondroitin, as well as omega-3; and taking medication to treat your pain if needed.

Motrin, Advil, topical NSAIDs, and acetaminophen have all stopped working for my OA knee pain. What's my next step?

There are actually still several very good treatment choices for you. You could try Lidoderm, tramadol, duloxetine, or opioid medication to see if these can give you good pain relief without bad side effects. Also, you can try hyaluronic acid joint injections. If these fail too, and your pain and disability are severe, you may be a candidate for knee replacement surgery.

Anticipating RA:
A Patient's Story

I always dreaded getting this type of arthritis. I watched my grandmother and mother slowly become crippled by the condition. By the time they reached their mid-seventies, their fingers were all deformed and they could barely move them. Now that I am forty-five, I've noticed pain and stiffness in my finger joints, especially in the morning. I take OTC Motrin with good relief, but I really don't want to become like my grandmom and mom. Luckily, my doctor mentioned there are now revolutionary types of medications that can slow the progression of the disease, which were not available to them.

RA treatment has two major goals: to alleviate the associated symptoms of pain and stiffness, and to prevent long-term damage and disability.

Although RA is not yet curable, many treatments—most of them medications—can have significant beneficial effects on both the pain and the symptoms of OA as well as preventing joint destruction.

- ✓ Disease-modifying antirheumatic drugs (DMARDs)
- ✓ Other medications-for-pain
- ✓ PT
- ✓ Weight loss
- ✓ Surgery

Symptoms of RA

You have RA, which is serious but not always debilitating. Unlike most other chronic pain conditions the symptoms of RA wax and wane, with symptom-free periods. These symptom-free periods (remissions) can last weeks, months, or for some people, even years. When the disease is active and inflammation is present, there is significant stiffness and pain, especially in the morning and after periods of inactivity of the involved joints.

The most common joints affected by RA are the fingers, hands, and feet, although any joint can be involved. Most often, more than one joint is affected, and joint movement is typically painful and limited. If the covering membrane of the joint is also involved, the joint becomes swollen, tender, warm, and stiff. During an active phase of RA, patients often complain of a low-grade fever, general tiredness, and loss of appetite. With chronic RA, there may be deformity and significant disability, and patients are at risk for developing osteoporosis.

About 10 percent of people with RA will have other organs affected by RA. In some of these people, the skin is involved, and patients will develop rheumatoid nodules under the skin over the joints. When the lung is involved, patients will develop abnormal scarring and fibrous tissue in their lungs, causing shortness of breath and a dry, hacking cough. The cardiovascular system is also at risk; people with RA are somewhat more prone to arthrosclerosis, heart attack, inflammation of the membrane covering the heart (pericarditis), and stroke.

RA Is Less Common Than OA, But More Serious

Unlike OA, RA is an autoimmune disease, which means your immune system behaves incorrectly and attacks your joints. Because RA can attack other parts of your body, it is a more serious medical condition than OA. RA causes chronic inflammation in the joints, and often in the soft tissues (muscles, tendons, and ligaments) and skin. The lining of the joints, called the *synovial membrane*, can also become inflamed. Though RA causes destruction of the joint, there is no correlation between the symptoms of pain, stiffness, and swelling and the degree of joint damage. Although RA is a chronic illness, meaning it can last for years, patients may experience long periods without symptoms. However, RA is typically a progressive illness that has the potential to cause joint destruction and functional disability.

Who Gets RA?

Approximately two million Americans suffer from RA, and it is more common in females than males. All races are at the same risk for developing RA. Most often the disease starts between the ages of forty and sixty. There appears to be a genetic inheritance as RA does tend to run in families, but unlike eye color, the genetics of RA are complicated and not yet fully understood. Currently, it is believed that having certain inherited genes may make you more susceptible to having RA, but having these genes does not make it 100 percent guaranteed that you will develop RA at some point in your lifetime.

Get the Facts: Classified Stages of RA

Rheumatologists—specialists among arthritis doctors—often classify RA according to the following criteria:

- **Class I:** completely able to perform usual activities of daily living
- **Class II:** able to perform usual self-care and work activities, but limited in activities outside of work (such as playing sports or doing household chores)
- **Class III:** able to perform usual self-care activities, but limited in work and other activities
- **Class IV:** limited in ability to perform usual self-care, work, and other activities

Step-By-Step Treatment for RA

Depending on the severity of your RA symptoms, both in your joints and if present in other parts of your body, your doctor may prescribe special RA disease-modifying drugs (DMARDs). For your pain, you may first try some OTC drugs or prescription pain drugs. Also, all patients should try nondrug treatments, such as PT and exercise. Because the progression of RA is so different from person to person, your doctor will likely want to see you on a fairly regular basis to monitor how you are doing. For RA, you should probably find a good rheumatology doctor with whom you develop a good working relationship.

▼ **NORMAL JOINT (LEFT) VERSUS JOINT WITH RHEUMATOID ARTHRITIS (RIGHT)**

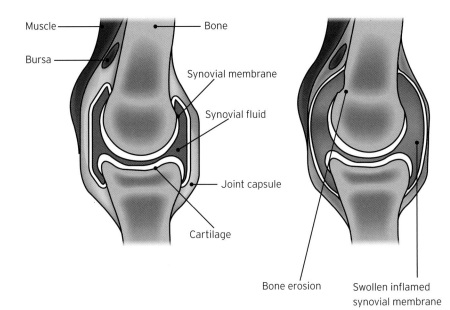

Muscle

Bone

Bursa

Synovial membrane

Synovial fluid

Joint capsule

Cartilage

Bone erosion

Swollen inflamed synovial membrane

DMARDs: Handle with Care

In 2008, the American College of Rheumatology published *Recommendations for the Use of Nonbiologic and Biologic DMARDs in RA*. These are quite complicated guidelines for doctors to follow, as there are many different scenarios to follow, depending on each patient's condition and other medical factors. Here, we briefly summarize their recommendations—but again, we must reiterate that if you have RA, you need to be evaluated and treated by a well-trained rheumatologist.

- Leflunomide (Arava) or methotrexate therapy should be prescribed for all RA patients, regardless of the duration of RA or the severity of symptoms.
- In new RA cases or those where symptoms are becoming more severe, an anti-TNF agent can be prescribed in conjunction with methotrexate therapy.
- Studies have shown the biologic DMARDs to be most effective when given in combination with methotrexate.
- Leflunomide, methotrexate, and biologic therapies should not be prescribed for RA patients with active bacterial infections, herpes zoster (shingles), hepatitis B or C, or tuberculosis in either the active or latent stage.
- RA patients with multiple sclerosis, lymphoma, or heart failure should not be given anti-TNF drugs.

METHOTREXATE: THE MOST FREQUENTLY PRESCRIBED DMARD FOR RA

For most doctors, methotrexate has become the first drug they prescribe for RA patients who they feel could benefit from a DMARD. Methotrexate interferes with the way cells utilize essential nutrients. In RA, it affects the ability of immune cells to secrete inflammatory chemicals, and thereby reduces inflammation.

Methotrexate has several good qualities:

- Rapid onset of action as compared to other DMARDs (six to eight weeks)
- Works well for most patients, with limited side effects
- Easy to use
- Inexpensive

In addition, one study found that when comparing different DMARDs, the majority of patients continue to take methotrexate after five years, longer than other DMARDs, due to its efficacy and tolerability.

The most common side effect of methotrexate is nausea, but luckily for most patients, this goes away in less than a week. For those who continue to have nausea, antinausea pills are available that seem to work for most people.

What's New: DMARDs Go After the Disease

Luckily for the current generation of RA sufferers, a new category of anti-RA drugs, called DMARDs, has succeeded in working directly against the abnormal RA process.

What are DMARDs? DMARDs are a critical part of RA treatment. By definition, DMARDs are drugs that can reduce the rate of bone and cartilage damage in RA-afflicted joints. It is possible for these drugs to stop RA in its tracks, resulting in prolonged remissions. Because damage from RA is permanent, most experts now recommend these drugs be started sooner rather than later, before damage begins.

What types of DMARDs are available? DMARDs are subdivided into older nonbiologic drugs and newer biologic DMARDs, which have revolutionized the treatment of RA. The tumor necrosis factor (TNF) blockers, for example, are biologic DMARDs that prevent the TNF messenger protein from activating the inflammation process in an RA joint. All DMARDs are very potent and can have serious side effects; they should be prescribed by a knowledgeable and experienced doctor, usually a rheumatologist.

Benefits versus Risks of TNF DMARDs

We all know that our choices in life involve weighing potential big upsides alongside risks that bad stuff may happen; a lot of Americans recently learned this hard lesson when betting in the stock market or real estate. This is the case with new TNF blockers. These "miracle drugs" have the potential for dramatic positive results in about 70 percent of RA patients, but they also have significant potential for medical risks. The two most common serious risks are infections including tuberculosis and lymphoma. Most recently, the FDA added warnings about an increase in cancers in children using these drugs, including lymphomas, leukemias, melanomas, and solid organ cancers. Thus, we recommend that all of our RA patients seek counsel with an experienced rheumatologist. It truly is a hard decision, especially in early cases of RA where symptoms are minimal or easily treated with simple analgesics, because when RA progresses, damage to the joints and other body organs is irreversible.

HOW DO TNF DMARDS WORK?

The tumor necrosis factor-alpha (TNF) blocker drugs—etanercept (Enbrel), infliximab (Remicade), and adalimumab (Humira)—prevent the messenger protein TNF from turning on cells in the joint that release inflammatory chemicals. TNF is produced naturally by white blood cells in the blood and joint, and can cause joint damage. Thus, TNF blockers can significantly prevent RA-related joint destruction and improve pain and disability.

Other Medications to Treat RA Pain

In addition to DMARDs, several medications are suggested for treating the pain and stiffness of RA that have no effect on the underlying disease. These are the same medical treatments suggested for OA pain, so we will only briefly discuss them here.

TOPICAL NSAIDS PENETRATE THE SKIN WITH MEDICINE

Topical NSAIDs have only recently been approved by the FDA for OA pain, and they come in solution, gel, and patch forms. The drugs, such as Pennsaid, Voltaren Gel, and Flector Patch, deliver the same pain-relieving chemicals as classic NSAID pills, but penetrate the skin over the painful joint without significantly altering blood levels. None of these drugs have been studied for RA pain, nor are they FDA-approved to treat the pain and symptoms of RA, although theoretically, they may help some patients' pain.

ACETAMINOPHEN WORKS WELL, WHEN TAKEN CORRECTLY

Studies have shown that this OTC drug gives many RA patients good pain relief without side effects. However, use this drug with caution; acetaminophen overuse is the number-one cause of liver damage and liver transplants in the United States!

NSAIDS/COX-2 INHIBITORS REDUCE INFLAMMATION

These drugs reduce joint inflammation and have direct pain-relieving actions in the spinal cord. When taken in recommended doses, they can be very helpful. However, if consumed too frequently or at too high a dose, they can cause potentially serious side effects, even with OTC preparations such as Motrin, Advil, and Aleve.

LIDOCAINE PATCH 5% (LIDODERM) DECREASES PAIN SIGNALS

Lidocaine has been shown in several studies to provide good pain relief and no serious side effects when delivered via a patch applied to the skin overlying an OA joint, but has not been studied for RA. Experts believe the lidocaine diffuses into the joint to decrease the signals coming from joint pain nerves. Lidocaine patch 5% is not FDA-approved to treat RA pain, nor has it been studied in RA patients, but based on some studies showing relief in OA joints, this drug may also help to alleviate some patients' RA pain.

TRAMADOL MAY ALSO WORK FOR RA PAIN

Tramadol works on two different pain pathways in the brain and spinal cord: those that use natural opioids and those that use the neurochemicals norepinephrine and serotonin. Being a general overall pain reliever and being shown to work for OA pain, tramadol should also work well for some people with RA pain.

DULOXETINE (CYMBALTA) HELPS WITH KNEE PAIN

Recently, several good scientific studies have demonstrated that duloxetine relieves the pain of knee OA, and therefore will be effective for some patients with RA pain, although it is not FDA-approved for this indication. Duloxetine works on neurochemicals in the brain and spinal cord that are involved in both pain and depression, norepinephrine and serotonin. However, like many antidepressants that work for pain, duloxetine alleviates pain even if the patient is not depressed.

OPIOIDS ARE RESERVED FOR SEVERE RA CONDITIONS

Because opioids can work for all types of pain, the same rules that are used to treat OA pain should be used to treat RA pain. These drugs work in the pain regions of the brain and spinal cord, where there are natural opioid-like neurochemicals. In addition, these drugs may also have an effect locally in inflamed tissues, such as an inflamed joint.

In our opinion, as when using opioids to treat any chronic pain condition, opioids should not be prescribed as first-line medications, but they should be used for hard-to-treat RA patients with moderate to severe refractory pain.

Nonmedication Treatments For RA Pain
EXERCISE AND PT MAINTAIN MOBILITY

As with OA, regular exercise of the involved arthritic joints is strongly recommended for RA sufferers. This will maintain joint mobility, as well as strengthen the muscles that support and move the joint. You should choose an exercise that you find enjoyable, and most importantly, do it regularly, whether it is walking, bicycling, swimming, or just moving your RA joints through their usual range of motion.

Your overall exercise program should involve the following elements:

- Stretching/range of motion of your RA joints
- Stretching should be done passively, meaning you gently stretch the muscles, tendons, and ligaments around your joints. This should be done every day for five to seven repetitions, increasing to ten repetitions per day. It's important to stretch in a slow, steady manner without bouncing or stretching to the point of pain, and to breathe regularly.
  - First relax your hand, and straighten your fingers, putting them close together. Then bend your middle and top finger joints while keeping your wrist and knuckles straight. Then slowly straighten your fingers (see figure a).
  - Start with your fingers spread as far apart as you can. Then gently make a fist with your thumb wrapped around your fingers. There's no need to make a tight fist, as the goal of this exercise is to move your fingers, not to eventually punch someone! Then return your fingers and hand to the original position (see figure b).
  - Hold your fingers straight, and then spread them apart as wide as you can. Hold them in that position for a few seconds, and then slowly relax them and bring them together. Finally, return to the original position (see figure c).
- Strengthening exercises
  - Isometric exercises are recommended, especially when painful joints limit your movement. The joint and muscles do not move, but are worked against an immovable force or are held in the same position while being opposed by resistance.

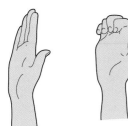

▲ Figure a

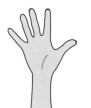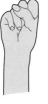

▲ Figure b

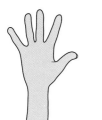

▲ Figure c

- You should contract the muscle being exercised with maximum force and hold it for three to six seconds. Start with two to three repetitions, and slowly progress by increasing to ten repetitions. You should do these exercises three times per week.
- Aerobic exercise
  - Find a low-impact activity that reduces the amount of weight you put on your OA joints (e.g., swimming, biking, or rowing). It really doesn't matter what form of exercise you do, as long as you do it regularly and move your joints. Just be sure you avoid exercises that put too much stress on your joints, and make sure you find shoes and insoles that provide good shock absorption.

AVOIDING CERTAIN FOODS MAY HELP

Some doctors and Web sites may recommend avoiding nightshade foods, such as potatoes, tomatoes, peppers, and eggplant, but no studies have proven this to be effective. (The name "nightshade" reportedly comes from the fact that most of these vegetables are believed to grow in the nighttime.) However, there's no harm in evaluating this for yourself to see if you begin to see a pattern after you eat such foods.

FISH OIL REDUCES INFLAMMATION

Fish oil supplements have been shown to have an anti-inflammatory effect, but their role in helping RA has not been demonstrated. However, because fish oil capsules have no side effects, can help with other chronic conditions, and may help with RA, we do recommend their daily use. A study has not shown the optimal dose, but based on current knowledge, we recommend 2–4 grams per day of omega-3 fatty acids.

WEIGHT LOSS DECREASES PAIN

Overburdening your inflamed RA joints with extra pounds can only cause more inflammation, damage, pain, and stiffness. We urge you to get rid of your unnecessary weight. You will have fewer RA symptoms and be much healthier overall.

Examination Findings: Inflammation and Deformity

After asking you questions about your symptoms, a doctor will closely examine your joints, especially in your fingers and hands, for inflammation and deformity. Your doctor will also look at your skin for rheumatoid nodules around your joints, as well as other parts of the body for inflammation. Because the symptoms and examination findings come and go with RA, your doctor will likely want to examine you several times and ask that when you have worsening joint symptoms you make an urgent appointment so that he or she can examine you during an acute episode of symptoms.

1987 Criteria for the Classification of Acute Rheumatoid Arthritis

A patient must have at least four of the seven criteria in the following list. Criteria 1 through 4 must have been present for at least six weeks.

1. **Morning stiffness.** Morning stiffness in and around the joints, lasting at least one hour before maximal improvement

2. **Arthritis of three or more joint areas.** At least three joint areas simultaneously have had soft tissue swelling or fluid. The fourteen possible joint areas include the hand, finger, wrist, elbow, knee, ankle, and foot joints

3. **Arthritis of hand joints.** At least one area swollen (as defined in criterion 2) in a wrist or finger

4. **Symmetric arthritis.** Involvement of the same joint areas (as defined in criterion 2) on both sides of the body

5. **Rheumatoid nodules** Subcutaneous (under the skin) nodules

6. **Serum rheumatoid factor.** Abnormal blood test showing elevated serum rheumatoid factor

7. **Radiographic (X-ray) changes.** X-ray changes typical of RA in hand and wrist

OCCUPATIONAL THERAPY PROVIDES INDEPENDENCE

If RA joints become damaged and debilitating, an evaluation by an occupational therapist is strongly recommended. This person can teach you certain tricks to improve your daily activities or, if needed, recommend certain devices such as canes, toilet seat raisers, and jar grippers that can make your life more enjoyable and give you back some independence.

SURGERY MAKES A DRAMATIC DIFFERENCE

For severely debilitated and damaged RA joints of the knee and hip, joint replacement surgery can be a miracle treatment. Although this surgery sounds dramatic, it is actually a fairly common treatment today. Many surgeons who specialize in joint replacement can perform several such surgeries every day successfully.

Diagnosing RA

The current diagnostic criteria were published in 1987 by the American College of Rheumatology (see the sidebar "1987 Criteria for the Classification of Acute Rheumatoid Arthritis"). Although initially written for clinical trial and research purposes, these criteria are commonly used today by doctors. As you can see, a doctor can make the diagnosis of RA based mostly on your symptoms and what he or she sees when examining certain joints in your hands, fingers, wrists, elbows, and feet. Findings on blood tests and X-rays can help confirm the diagnosis.

DIAGNOSTIC BLOOD TESTS FOR RA

The "diagnostic" blood test looks for rheumatoid factor (RF), which is an antibody. However, if the test comes back negative—that is, with no RF in your blood—it does not mean you do not have RA. Actually, about 15 percent of patients with RA do not have RF, but with time most RA patients eventually have evidence of RF in their blood. On the other hand, having a positive RF test doesn't necessarily mean you have RA, since other conditions can also cause RF in the blood.

X-RAY TESTS FOR RA

Old-fashioned X-rays of your hands and other affected joints are typically performed every year to provide a baseline and track your progression. As with the blood test, in early stages of RA the X-rays may be completely normal. However, over time the X-rays of the affected joints of patients will show swelling of soft tissues. And as RA progresses, bony erosions will be seen in the joints.

RA Explained

RA is an autoimmune disease. Autoimmune diseases are conditions caused by a person's immune system when it begins to abnormally attack the body. In RA, antibodies attack the synovial membranes that line the joints. It is not known why this occurs or what triggers it, but RA is now believed to be a genetically inherited disorder. RA is a systemic illness, and therefore may involve not only the joints, but also other organs and tissues throughout the body.

The chemical TNF seems to play a large role in the development and progression of RA. TNF is a cytokine, a protein secreted by immune cells. When TNF is released by immune cells, it results in inflammation and begins a significant inflammatory response.

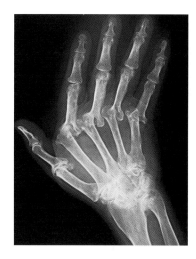

▲ X-ray of a hand with rheumatoid arthritis

What's New: Positive Antibody Tests for RA

In addition to the RF test, other antibody blood tests have recently become available to better detect which patients have RA, especially if all of the antibody blood tests are positive.

What do these tests find? These other tests look for the presence of anticitrullinated protein antibodies, which are found in about 70 percent of patients with RA, but rarely are present in other conditions. Other antibodies sometimes tested for in the blood are anti-CCP (cyclic citrullinated peptide) and anti-MCV assay (antibodies against mutated citrullinated vimentin).

The Natural Course of RA

RA varies greatly from person to person. However, for most RA sufferers, the disease is progressive. With the advent of DMARDs, significant strides have been made in slowing the progression of RA in most patients.

If left untreated, RA will progress and will slowly cause disability in the involved joints. Also, if other organs or body parts, such as the eyes, lung, heart, blood vessels, or nerves, are afflicted with RA, other significant health issues may arise. Thus, unlike most conditions with chronic pain (and the ones we describe in this book), RA can spread and involve other organs, and so it is critically important that RA patients have constant medical follow-up and monitoring.

CONCLUSION: BREAKTHROUGHS OFFER HOPE FOR RA TREATMENT

Unlike the other chronic pain conditions we discuss in this book, RA is a serious progressive disorder that, if left untreated, will result in critical disability for most patients, although the rate of progression can be extremely slow for some RA patients. The good news is that breakthroughs in treatment can significantly reduce the rate of progression and alleviate much pain and disability in most RA patients.

My doctor recommends I immediately start DMARD treatment, even though I can live with my RA symptoms. What should I do?

Not an easy question to answer since this is not a "black and white" question. This is an individual decision. Currently though, many RA experts are recommending that all patients with definite RA should be treated with DMARDs, since once the disease starts the damage that it does is irreversible. However, your fear of starting these powerful medicines are justified too, since they are associated with some potentially serious side effects. We recommend discussing the options with your doctors, your family, and others with RA.

My mother had RA. Will I definitely get it when I'm older?

No. Though the chances are better than 50/50 you will eventually have RA, some things cannot be predicted, such as at what age you may develop symptoms of RA, how severe a case of RA you may get (less or more serious than your mother), and if you develop RA what the rate of progression will be.

CHAPTER 4

Repressing Neuropathic Pain

Many medications can have a profound effect on neuropathic pain.

the PRESCRIPTION for NEUROPATHIC PAIN

If you've been reading the other chapters in this book, you'll notice a difference in the prescription for treating most neuropathic pain.

Except for one specific type of neuropathic pain, Reflex Sympathetic Dystrophy/Complex Regional Pain Syndrome (RSD/CRPS), physical therapy (PT) or exercise is not as important as medications and psychological treatments. The reasons are twofold: Many patients find medicines that significantly relieve their pain intensity; and there is often little to be gained by nonmedication treatments that aim to relieve neuropathic pain. People with some types of neuropathic pain are at high risk for developing depression and anxiety, which should be treated separately by a psychiatrist.

✓ Medications
✓ Psychiatry (if you are depressed, are anxious, or have symptoms of post-traumatic stress disorder [PTSD])

Tingling and Painful Toes:
A Patient's Story

I'm a fifty-five-year-old man who has had pain for about three years now. At first, I began to notice a funny tingling in my toes, sort of like a pins-and-needles sensation. Then it gradually became a sharp pain in all of my toes. In the past year or so, the pain has spread to the rest of my feet on both sides. And over the past few months, I have begun to notice pain up to my calves on both sides. Also, the pain is more severe and disabling. It's a constant, intense aching, and sometimes I get these horrible sharp electric shocks after walking. On most days now I have trouble wearing socks or shoes because the skin on my feet gets very sensitive, like raw skin. My feet also sometimes feel icy cold and like they are blocks of wood. I sleep poorly due to the pain, and my wife says I've gotten pretty irritable. She calls me a grouchy old man, and I'm only fifty-five!

What's New: Medications for Peripheral Neuropathic Pain

Over the past decade, many new medications have been developed and shown to be safe and effective in treating all peripheral neuropathic pain conditions.

What kinds of medications are they? These medicatons fall into several categories: topical drugs, antiseizure medications, antidepressant medications, and opioids. All of these are truly medications for pain, though initially they may have been developed by a pharmaceutical company to treat other types of medical conditions, such as seizures and depression.

Do they help all kinds of neuropathic pain? Although many have been approved by the FDA to treat only certain peripheral nerve pain conditions, most experts believe, as we do, that all of these medications may be help-ful in treating all types of peripheral neuropathic pain conditions, and in addition, central neuropathic pain.

A Case of the Nerves

Anytime there is damage to a nerve in the body, chronic nerve pain or what is commonly referred to as *neuropathic pain* can result. Neuropathic pain is divided into peripheral neuropathic pain and central neuropathic pain, depending on which part of the nervous system is damaged: the peripheral nervous system (peripheral nerves) or the central nervous system (brain and spinal cord).

In this chapter, we will describe the three most common peripheral neuropathic pain conditions: painful polyneuropathy (which includes diabetic neuropathy), postherpetic neuralgia (PHN, also known as chronic shingles pain), and RSD/CRPS.

Peripheral neuropathic pain most often develops after damage or inflammation to the peripheral nerves—in particular, the small nerves that normally provide sensory information from your skin, muscles, and organs. Like a damaged electrical wire, when these nerves get injured or inflamed they basically "short-circuit," sending abnormal pain signals to the spinal cord and then on up to the brain, even if no painful event is occurring (such as being stabbed by a knife or burned by a match).

▶ Note how extensive the peripheral nervous system is.

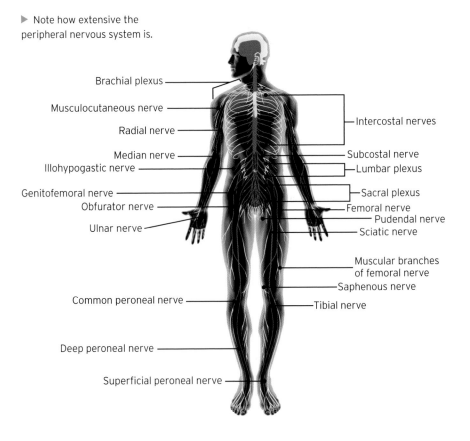

Brachial plexus

Musculocutaneous nerve

Radial nerve

Median nerve

Illohypogastric nerve

Genitofemoral nerve

Obfurator nerve

Ulnar nerve

Intercostal nerves

Subcostal nerve

Lumbar plexus

Sacral plexus

Femoral nerve

Pudendal nerve

Sciatic nerve

Muscular branches of femoral nerve

Saphenous nerve

Common peroneal nerve

Tibial nerve

Deep peroneal nerve

Superficial peroneal nerve

Medications to Treat Neuropathic Pain

For most patients with neuropathic pain (excluding RSD/CRPS), medication is usually the only treatment that is required. However, it's important to realize that individual variability exists for each drug. In other words, even though patients may have the same diagnosis, they will vary in their response to any particular drug. Patients will experience different degrees of pain relief and side effects at different doses; there is no magic pill or dose for every patient with neuropathic pain. The doctor needs to try one medication at a time, at a low dose, and gradually increase it, depending on how the patient responds. Some patients may require a combination of several different drugs to obtain the best balance of pain relief and side effects. We know it can be frustrating for patients, but your doctor must use a trial-and-error method. The good news is that there are many different types of drugs to try, so hang in there and let your doctor find the right one(s) for you.

The following list is recommended by panels of leading neuropathic pain experts around the world, several of which we have served on. It is important to realize that all of the medications on these lists specifically work for chronic nerve pain conditions. Though they all act differently and in different locations in the nervous system, they all have been shown in studies to significantly help some people with a variety of chronic neuropathic pain. However, unfortunately, none have been shown to cure the pain. They all must be used daily and continually for them to work.

LIDOCAINE PATCH 5% (LIDODERM) LOWERS THE PAIN VOLUME

Although lidocaine patch 5% is currently FDA-approved to treat only PHN, several studies have shown it to be effective in alleviating the pain of other peripheral neuropathic conditions, including diabetic neuropathy and other polyneuropathies, as well as stump and neuroma pain. The lidocaine from the patch penetrates through the skin, finds its way to the abnormally active peripheral nerves that are signaling the pain, and reduces the frequency and intensity of these abnormal pain signals. The formulation of the lidocaine patch is unique and results in pain relief without causing skin numbness ("analgesia without anesthesia"); thus, replacing it with other forms of topical lidocaine will not have the same effect. The FDA-approved dosing for lidocaine patch 5% is to use up to three patches at a time applied to the painful area twelve hours on and then twelve hours off. However, many studies have been published that show it is safe to use up to four patches at a time, keeping them on for twenty-four hours and then putting on new patches.

What's New: Punch-Skin Biopsy for Peripheral Polyneuropathy

A relatively new type of test is being performed that is fairly benign yet can be very helpful for doctors in diagnosing certain kinds of neuropathy: the punch-skin biopsy.

How does it work? The doctor uses a pen-like device to take 0.12-inch (3 mm) circular slivers of skin (usually two or three) from the distal leg. The doctor then examines these skin pieces under a microscope using specific stains that allow him or her to visualize different types of nerves. There are no bad side effects, and the biopsy sites heal within two weeks without any scarring.

What does it diagnose? Punch-skin biopsies are now most useful for rare neuropathies in which it is difficult for a doctor to make a diagnosis. Also, some university doctors are using it as a prognostic tool to evaluate how rapidly the neuropathy will progress.

73

What's New: Topical Analgesics for Peripheral Neuropathic Pain

Developing drugs that are applied to the skin and work only in the peripheral nervous system without producing significant blood levels could, at least theoretically, result in good pain relief with minimal side effects.

Are these in development? Scientists (such as Dr. Argoff) and drug developers (such as Dr. Galer) are searching for neurochemicals and inflammatory chemicals in peripheral nerves, skin, and muscles that play a role in peripheral neuropathic pain conditions (and other pain conditions). Several new potential targets include a chemical called NMDA, inflammatory cytokines, opioids, and cannabinoids (yes, naturally occurring marijuana-like substances).

(continued)

PREGABALIN (LYRICA) AND GABAPENTIN (NEURONTIN): BOTH GOOD

These drugs, from the same chemical family (gabapentinoids), were first designed as antiseizure medications. Gabapentin is FDA-approved to treat only PHN. Pregabalin is FDA-approved to treat painful diabetic polyneuropathy and PHN. Both gabapentin and pregabalin work on the alpha-2-delta receptor (in the calcium channels of nerves found in the brain and spinal cord), which are believed to play a role in the pain system. Both gabapentin and pregabalin have been shown in studies of nerve injuries in animals to work on pain directly on injured peripheral nerves as well.

These are probably the best-studied drugs for all types of neuropathic pain. Because they are effective and better tolerated than most other oral drugs, they are also considered a first-line treatment by world experts (including us).

As compared to gabapentin, pregabalin may have some advantages. Pregabalin typically requires less time to find an effective dose. Also, some studies have found that patients who fared poorly with gabapentin, due to either poor pain relief or bad side effects, do well with pregabalin. However, gabapentin in now available as a generic drug, and therefore is usually much less expensive for patients.

DULOXETINE (CYMBALTA) RESTORES BALANCE

Duloxetine has been approved by the FDA to treat diabetic neuropathy pain. Other studies and experience have shown it to be effective for some people with other neuropathic pain conditions, such as PHN. This drug is a selective serotonin and norepinephrine reuptake inhibitor and is believed to work by restoring the balance of serotonin and norepinephrine in the brain and spinal cord. Some patients can have side effects with duloxetine, including nausea, fatigue, dizziness, and constipation.

TRICYCLIC ANTIDEPRESSANTS MAY HAVE BAD SIDE EFFECTS

None of the tricyclic antidepressants (TCAs) have an FDA-approved indication to treat any neuropathic pain disorder, although they are one of the oldest types of medications that have been used successfully. (The reason they don't have FDA approval to treat any neuropathic pain condition is because they became generic before it was realized they can treat nerve pain.) TCAs such as amitriptyline, nortriptyline, and desipramine have been shown in many studies to relieve the pain of diabetic polyneuropathy and PHN, whether or not a patient is depressed. These drugs also work on the brain and spinal cord chemicals serotonin and norepinephrine.

However, the TCAs often cause bad side effects in many pain patients. TCAs may cause severe dry mouth, constipation, sedation, thinking difficulties, and a decrease in blood pressure upon standing. There is also a rare risk of heart rhythm disturbance. Therefore, it is now recommended that all patients undergo an EKG before and during treatment with TCAs.

OPIOIDS OFFER MEANINGFUL RELIEF FOR SOME

About a decade ago, doctors (including us) were taught that opioids did not work for any type of neuropathic pain. Well, now we know better! Studies have shown that opioid medications, such as morphine, oxycodone, hydrocodone, and oxymorphone, can give some patients with neuropathic pain meaningful relief without intolerable side effects, and with no addiction (see chapter 8 for a discussion of opioid use).

Importantly, if you try one opioid medication and you don't experience good pain relief or you get bad side effects, it may be worthwhile to try another one. Studies have shown that just because you don't do well with one opioid doesn't necessarily mean you'll do badly with another.

THE RIGHT DOSE OF NARCOTIC-OPIOID DRUGS

For neuropathic pain, a long-acting opioid drug should be prescribed around the clock and not on an as-needed basis. The dose should be gradually increased to find the best daily dose, as is done with all of the other oral drugs. Short-acting opioids may also be prescribed for episodes of breakthrough pain on an as-needed basis.

DOES MARIJUANA HELP RELIEVE PAIN?

This is a very hot topic in both the scientific and legal worlds. Although strong scientific evidence shows that cannabinoid chemicals and receptors exist naturally in all parts of the nervous system—brain, spinal cord, and peripheral nerves—and that these natural chemicals appear to play some role in alleviating pain in animal studies, there is still no strong evidence that smoking marijuana will have a significant pain-relieving effect in people. That being said, it may be that this evidence is lacking only because good clinical trials have not been performed. We both have had patients who have told us (in confidence) that smoking marijuana has helped them. The jury is still out....

(What's New: continued)

How do they work? As mentioned, topical drugs are applied to and penetrate through the skin overlying the painful region, where they work directly on the injured or abnormally acting nerves, joints, and muscles. Depending on the drug being applied, the effect will vary. One interesting, very recent study found that the nonsteroidal anti-inflammatory drug diclofenac was shown in an animal model to have an effect on a distinct neurotransmitter, NMDA, which is known to be involved in certain neuropathic pain states. Thus, although the drug has not yet been studied in people with neuropathic pain (they are currently used to treat arthritis and musculoskeletal pain), this finding may suggest that topical diclofenac formulations also may be of benefit for certain peripheral neuropathic pain conditions.

What's New: Nutraceuticals for Peripheral Neuropathy

Three nutraceuticals you can buy in health food and vitamin stores have been found in studies to help certain types of neuropathy:

- **Acetyl-l-carnitine (ALC)** has been shown to improve neuropathy symptoms and even nerve function for diabetic neuropathy, chemotherapy-induced neuropathy, and HIV neuropathy, when 2–3 grams are taken per day. ACL seems to work best in patients who have had neuropathy for fewer than five years. ALC is believed to help the inner workings of the nerve.

- Similarly, the powerful antioxidant **alpha lipoic acid (ALA)** has been shown in studies of diabetic neuropathy to improve pain and other symptoms when given as intravenous infusions of 600 mg ALA for five days per week for fourteen treatments. One study evaluating ALA when taken orally as a pill found that the optimal dose is 600 mg per day for the treatment of symptomatic diabetic neuropathy.

(continued)

Nonmedication Therapies For Neuropathic Pain

REHABILITATION IS KEY FOR RSD/CRPS

An active physical/occupational therapy program is probably the most important element of treating RSD/CRPS. However, for all other neuropathic pain conditions, such a program usually is not of primary importance because PT and exercise do not have any effect on the underlying problem or help to relieve the pain. If, however, a patient is in poor physical condition due to the neuropathic pain, rehabilitative therapies may significantly improve the patient's ability to perform daily activities, and thus improve his or her quality of life.

SPINAL CORD STIMULATION INTERFERES WITH PAIN SIGNAL

Spinal cord stimulation employs a device that is surgically implanted in a patient so that a small electrical current can be applied to a specific area next to the spinal cord, which can interfere with the pain signal as it travels up to the brain. Some evidence suggests that spinal cord stimulation may work for some patients with RSD/CRPS in particular and perhaps in a small minority of patients with painful polyneuropathy.

NERVE BLOCKS FOR SOME RSD/CRPS PATIENTS

Nerve blocks are procedures in which a doctor uses a long needle to inject a numbing medication such as Novocain, or steroids into the damaged or abnormally functioning nerve(s). Nerve blocks have only a potential role for some patients with RSD/CRPS, and do not work for every RSD/CRPS patient. Nerve blocks should not be used as a mainstay of treatment for painful polyneuropathy or PHN because they most often do not work, and if they do, they will provide only short-term pain relief.

SURGERY IS NOT USUALLY AN OPTION

There is no role for surgery in the treatment of any neuropathic pain, except refractory carpal tunnel syndrome, and then only when the pain and other symptoms do not respond adequately to all nonsurgical treatments.

PSYCHIATRY FOR THE DEPRESSED AND ANXIOUS

If you are depressed or anxious, we recommend that you seek an evaluation and possible treatment from a psychologist or psychiatrist. Please read chapter 11 on psychological treatments for a detailed discussion of this topic.

REDUCE YOUR ADRENALINE AND YOUR PAIN

Stress management tools, including biofeedback, relaxation, imagery, and hypnosis, may all improve neuropathic pain to some degree, especially if the patient notices that stress worsens his or her pain. As we fully describe in chapter 17, stress is actually a biological state in which adrenaline is pumped into your bloodstream. Injured nerves that cause pain are often very sensitive to adrenaline, producing an increase in pain.

MULTIDISCIPLINARY PAIN CLINIC (MPC) TREATMENT

Treatment at an MPC is essential for most patients with RSD/CRPS. However, for other neuropathic pain treatments, such integrated care is necessary only if a patient continues to suffer with pain, disability, and psychological disturbances after appropriate trials of medication and individual psychological therapy have been conducted.

(What's New: continued)

- An encouraging study of the antioxidant **vitamin E** compared cancer patients who took 600 mg per day during chemotherapy and for three months after stopping chemotherapy, with the amount of neuropathy side effects to patients who did not receive any vitamin E. This study found a dramatic decrease in the number of patients who developed chemotherapy-induced neuropathy in those who took vitamin E.

What's New: Exercise and Diet in the Treatment of Diabetic Neuropathy

A recent study demonstrated that after twelve months of intensive exercise and strict diet, participants reported an improvement in diabetic neuropathy symptoms, as compared to those who had "standard" care. Patients decreased their weight by about 10 percent and exercised 150 minutes per week for twelve months. What's more, examination of the nerves using skin biopsies showed signs of nerve regrowth in the exercise-and-strict-diet patients. Once again, studies are showing the importance of exercise and diet in yet another condition!

Examination Findings: Painful Polyneuropathy

The loss of a patient's ability to feel sensations in his or her feet is the most important change a doctor will look for upon examination. The doctor should also find a stocking or stocking-and-glove pattern of the patient's ability to feel sensations. The doctor will test the patient's ability to feel light touch, vibration, pain, and sometimes warm and cold and will look for abnormal decreases in reflexes in the ankles and knee.

Symptoms of Painful Polyneuropathy (Including Diabetic Neuropathy)

Symptoms of painful polyneuropathy start in the toes and feet and may, in some patients, gradually rise to the calves and knees in a stocking pattern. The symptoms initially are most often in one foot and not the other, but with time both feet typically become involved. If symptoms move to the upper calf or knee, the person may also begin to notice pain or abnormal sensations in his or her fingers and hands, referred to as a *stocking-and-glove pattern*.

As with all neuropathic pain, a person may describe his or her pain using a variety of terms, such as burning, raw skin, sharp, electric-like, stabbing, deep aching, freezing cold, like walking on ground glass, and/or itchy. Some people with neuropathic pain also complain that their skin is extremely sensitive to touch (those of us in the pain business call this *allodynia*). Some patients may experience one type of pain quality and not another.

Pain may not always be the first symptom; a person with polyneuropathy may first describe unusual sensations, such as numbness, pins and needles, or a tingling sensation. Some patients with polyneuropathy never develop pain, but may have numbness, while others may only feel abnormal sensations (tingling, itching, etc.). It is not known why some people with polyneuropathy have pain and others do not.

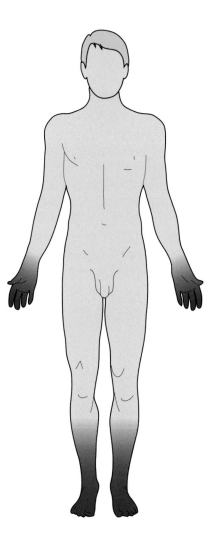

▲ Stocking and glove pattern of Polyneuropathy

Causes of Painful Polyneuropathy

The most common reasons peripheral nerves are injured, causing painful polyneuropathy, are:

- Diabetes
- Drugs, such as the chemotherapy drugs cisplatin, vincristine, and paclitaxel
- Alcoholism
- HIV/AIDS
- Idiopathic/unknown (in up to one-third of all neuropathies, the underlying cause remains unknown)

Diagnosing Painful Polyneuropathy

The diagnosis of painful polyneuropathy is based on history (what you tell the doctor about how it started and your symptoms) and examination findings. Specifically, the patient would describe pain (or numbness or tingling) that started in the toes and/or feet on both sides. Then, although not always, the symptoms would have gradually spread upward: toes to feet to calves to knees. Once the symptoms reach the upper calves or knees, some patients may begin to have pain or abnormal sensations in their fingers and hands.

Helpful Tests Outside The Lab
QUANTITATIVE SENSORY TESTING LOOKS AT NERVE FUNCTION

One way to test how the small nerve fibers are working is with Quantitative Sensory Testing (QST). This simple test assesses how patients feel temperature changes (warm and cold), which evaluates how the small nerves are working. Also, by testing the patient's ability to feel vibration, QST can also measure how well the large fibers are working. However, most doctors do not have a QST machine; some specialist neurologists may have one.

NERVE BIOPSY FOR MICROSCOPIC STUDY SHOULD RARELY BE DONE

Sometimes a doctor may recommend a nerve biopsy, which involves removing a piece of nerve and looking at it under a microscope. In our opinion, this should be done only if doctors cannot determine the cause of the neuropathy and if the neuropathy is spreading quickly. We have seen too many neuropathy patients who have had a nerve biopsy—not only was it not helpful in diagnosing or treating them, but it also caused a worsening pain problem. *Be cautious of nerve biopsies!*

Nerve Alert!

No Lab Tests Required
Unlike what some doctors may tell you (even neurologists), if your history and physical findings are consistent with the diagnosis of painful polyneuropathy, there is no need to perform any laboratory tests, including electrophysiological testing (electromyography [EMG] and nerve conduction [NCV]), to make the diagnosis. However, at times the pattern seen on these tests can help your doctor determine the cause of your polyneuropathy if he or she isn't sure.

If you get an EMG or NCV test, you should know that they can be very painful! These tests involve sticking thin needles into your muscles to see how the nerves connected to the muscles are working (EMG), and shocking your nerves to see how well they can conduct electricity and nerve signals (NCV).

Pain after Shingles:
A Patient's Story

I'm a 65-year-old proud grandmother. My pain problem
started three years ago when
my husband suddenly died. A
few months after his death, I
noticed a painful rash on the
right side of my chest, under
my breast, which spread to
my back. It looked like half of
a belt. It was quite painful. I
called my doctor and he knew
right away by how I described
it that it was shingles. Well, the
rash healed in a month or so,
but the pain never went away.
It's still pretty bad. I now have
two pain areas where the rash
was, one on one side of my
back and the other under my
right breast. There's always
a deep aching pain. What really upsets me is that I cannot
wear a bra because my skin
is so sensitive to anything
touching it. Also, at times I get
sharp pains in these bad spots.
At other times, the area feels
itchy, but scratching worsens
the pain. My doctor told me
there is nothing he can do for
me. Can you help me?

SKIN BIOPSY PROVIDES USEFUL INFORMATION

On the other hand, a fairly new procedure being used in some clinics is skin
biopsies (see "What's New: Punch-Skin Biopsy for Peripheral Polyneuropathy"),
which are relatively painless and can provide some potentially very useful
information, such as what types of nerves are damaged and to what degree
this damage has occurred.

Painful Polyneuropathy Explained

Several problems can happen to the sensory peripheral nerves that cause them
to become damaged or behave abnormally and result in polyneuropathy. Such
problems in the nerves can be caused by damage to the internal engine of the
nerve that helps it internalize needed nutrition, injury due to toxins in the body,
or perhaps viruses. Regardless of the underlying cause, the damaged peripheral
nerves do not get enough food and nutrients, and therefore can become sick,
starve, and may even die. Possible reasons for lack of nutrients in the nerve
can also include a poor blood supply, or perhaps the nerve itself is not able to
chemically digest the nutrients it needs to stay healthy.

Why does this type of neuropathy cause symptoms in a stocking or stocking-
and-glove pattern? It is believed that changes are dependent on the length of the
nerves, with the longer nerves being affected first. This is why the toes or feet are
the first place people feel their symptoms. Symptoms start there and then may
gradually move into the calves and knees, and then possibly into the fingers and
hands. This stocking-and-glove pattern is thought to be due to the fact that the
length of the nerves from the knee to the spine is approximately the same length
as from the fingers to the spine. As you'll learn in chapter 14, the sensory nerves
send their information about skin sensation to the spinal cord, where it then travels up to the brain.

For some types of painful polyneuropathy, the underlying cause can be treated
to help reduce or even eliminate the neuropathy. For instance, improved glucose
(sugar) control in diabetics has been shown to decrease pain and perhaps reduce
the progression of neuropathy. Alcohol, a toxin to peripheral nerves, should be
discontinued in patients with neuropathy. Also, if certain drugs are causing the
neuropathy, such as chemotherapy, stopping the drugs can reverse the nerve
damage so that chemotherapy neuropathies most often can resolve over time.

The Natural Course of Painful Polyneuropathy

Not everyone who develops a polyneuropathy will eventually have all of his or her hands, fingers, calves, feet, and toes affected with pain and other symptoms. In fact, most patients' symptoms stay only in their toes and feet. Also, the rate in which the polyneuropathy symptoms spread (if they spread at all) differs from person to person. It may take several decades or only several months, although this is very rare. For most people with more common forms of polyneuropathy, such as diabetic neuropathy, the spread occurs over many years, especially if the diabetes is under control and properly treated.

Symptoms Of Postherpetic Neuralgia (Chronic Shingles Pain)

You have PHN, a chronic pain that persists after the rash and blisters of acute shingles have healed. Although shingles and PHN can occur anywhere on the body, by far the most common places on the body for PHN are the chest and forehead; it rarely occurs on the arms and legs. PHN only occurs exactly where the shingles rash was.

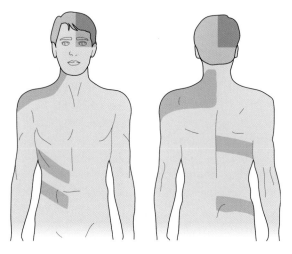

▲ Shingles (herpes zoster)–the most common locations affected

What's New: Insights into the Cause of Chemo Neuropathy

Over the past several years, a famous pain scientist, Gary Bennett Ph.D., has been studying chemotherapy-induced neuropathy using new animal models. Dr. Bennett's findings strongly suggest that some types of chemotherapy can negatively affect a certain part of the nerve cell, the mitochondria.

What do the mitochondria do?
The mitochondria are present in every living cell and are very important for cell survival and normal functioning. The mitochondria are basically the "energy factory" of each cell. So, when the mitochondria are sick, the cell will not be able to keep all of the normal ions (salts) inside versus outside the cell, which can result in abnormal signaling of pain from the damaged nerve cell.

Is the damage permanent?
Luckily, with most forms of chemotherapy this damage is not permanent; the mitochondria can again become healthy, and over time, the neuropathy can improve. Some ongoing studies are now evaluating drugs that keep mitochondria healthy to see if they can prevent and treat chemotherapy-induced neuropathies.

What's New: The Shingles Vaccine

In May 2006, the FDA approved a shingles vaccine (Zostavax) for adults age sixty and older.

Should everyone get it? People with conditions that weaken the immune system, such as lymphoma or leukemia, or who take drugs that weaken the immune system, including steroids, arthritis disease-modifying antirheumatic drugs (DMARDs), or chemotherapy, should not be given this vaccine.

Will the vaccine prevent shingles or PHN? The shingles vaccine does not guarantee that you won't get shingles. The studies did show that your risk of getting shingles is lowered by 51 percent and that if you do get shingles, your risk of getting PHN is reduced by 67 percent. If you do get shingles, it is likely that the pain you experience will be of decreased severity and duration. But like most things in life, nothing is guaranteed.

What are the side effects? The most common side effects of the shingles vaccine are redness, pain, tenderness, and swelling at the injection site, and headaches. Also, a major unanswered question is how long the vaccine's effects last. Studies are currently evaluating whether booster injections will be needed.

A PHN patient may describe the pain using a variety of terms, the most common being burning, raw skin; sharp; electric-like; deep; and achy. Unlike other neuropathic pain conditions, PHN patients may also complain of abnormal itching sensations. A very bothersome and common problem for most PHN patients is severe skin sensitivity (allodynia). Many folks with PHN are unable to wear clothing over their affected region because it is so sensitive to touch.

Although not very common, some patients describe the muscles in the PHN region as being weaker and flabbier, losing muscle tone. Psychological problems, especially depression, are common among PHN patients.

Once you hit 55 years of age, and then especially 65, the chance of getting shingles increases dramatically, and the risk of shingles turning into long-term PHN rises significantly as well. In addition to advanced age, other risk factors for developing PHN after shingles include severe pain during shingles, an underlying polyneuropathy, and significant depression or anxiety at the time of the shingles breakout.

REDUCING THE RISK OF GETTING PHN

Can anything reduce the chances of getting PHN after shingles? Starting antiviral medication, such as acyclovir, valacyclovir, and famciclovir, within a few days of rash onset can significantly reduce the chances of getting PHN. Also, the FDA has approved a shingles vaccine given to adults that has been shown in one study to reduce the chances of both getting shingles and developing PHN after shingles.

Diagnosing PHN

The diagnosis of PHN is actually quite simple; the patient has a history of shingles and continued pain in the same skin region. Therefore, no laboratory tests are usually needed to make the diagnosis of PHN.

PHN Explained

Unlike a lot of other chronic pain conditions, the exact cause of PHN is known. The disease process that can eventually cause PHN begins in childhood with chickenpox, caused by the varicella zoster virus, one of the herpes viruses. After the skin rash from chickenpox heals, the virus travels from the skin into the sensory nerves and then into a bundle of nerves next to the spinal cord (dorsal root ganglia), where the virus lives in hibernation, usually for decades.

Then, usually many decades later, the virus reemerges and begins to multiply within this nerve bundle. The virus then travels along the peripheral nerve back to the skin, where it causes the typical shingles rash. Unlike chickenpox, shingles always occurs on only one side of the body and in a belt-like fashion. The medical term for this is *acute herpes zoster.*

A decrease in a particular component of the immune system, called *cell-mediated immunity*, is what allows the virus to reawaken. Most often, the reason for the decrease in this component of the immune system is simply old age and/or stress. Probably one of the most common scenarios is when shingles develops in an elderly person who has recently had a major stressful life event, such as a major illness, surgery, or the death or illness of a loved one (as in our earlier story). Another possible medical reason for this reduction in the immune system is the use of drugs that decrease immunity, such as steroids or chemotherapy.

When the varicella zoster virus reawakens, it results in a severe inflammatory response and causes damage to the bundle of nerves where it has been living. Also, as it travels along the peripheral nerves to the skin, it can cause severe damage to these nerves as well. We think of it like the old arcade game Pac-Man, where the virus gobbles up nerve tissue as it moves from the nerve to the skin. Thus, PHN is caused by damage to peripheral nerves.

The Natural Course of PHN

Even though it is assumed that all patients with an acute shingles rash have had some degree of nerve damage, the vast majority of people who get shingles do not go on to develop PHN. It is not known why most shingles patients have a gradual reduction and eventual complete elimination of pain, whereas some unlucky people continue to have pain for months or even years. Most people experience their worst pain during the acute shingles rash period, and then, over the next few months, it gradually resolves. Within three to six months, most ex-shingles patients have no or very little pain.

For people who have PHN pain for more than six months, the pain may gradually reduce over several years. However, the potential for long-term chronic pain is greatest if the PHN pain continues for one year.

After the shingles rash has healed, the skin area may have a deep white discoloration and some scarring. When doctors examine the PHN skin area, they often find changes in sensation. Some PHN areas may have numbness and loss of sensation, and other areas can be extremely painful to light touch. Often in the same patient, skin patches of decreased and increased sensation are found right next to each other.

What's New: Treatments for PHN

Several drugs have been approved by the FDA to treat PHN, and many more have been proven effective.

What are they and how do they work? The first drug approved by the FDA specifically to treat the pain of PHN was the lidocaine patch 5% (Lidoderm), which acts locally to calm the damaged pain nerves but doesn't numb them. Subsequently, other drugs that have obtained FDA approval for PHN include gabapentin (Neurontin) and pregabalin (Lyrica), which are taken orally and are believed to work on the alpha-2-delta receptor found in the calcium channels of the nerves in the brain and spinal cord, and peripheral nerves. However, it is still not known how this alpha-2-delta interaction helps relieve nerve pain.

What are the side effects? Because lidocaine patch 5% works locally on the nerves under the skin where it is applied and doesn't cause any significant drug blood levels, the most common potential side effect is skin rash, which for most is a very minor problem. The most common side effects for gabapentin and pregabalin are tiredness, trouble concentrating, and nausea.

83

Hot, Cold, and Alien:
A Patient's Story

I am a thirty-one-year-old woman. About six months ago, I sprained my ankle playing softball. I sprained the same ankle several times before, but this time it just seemed different. When it first happened, I felt a sharp pain from my ankle into my foot. The pain has never left the foot or ankle. Over the first month, the foot became very cold and had a lot of swelling, with some burning pains and sensations of heat in the foot and ankle. The pain is now mostly a deep ache. I also still get burning pain when the foot becomes cold. I am unable to put a sock or shoe on because my foot is so sensitive to anything that touches it; even my bed sheets can cause a searing pain. The foot sometimes starts to sweat profusely when no other part of my body is sweating. Also, and this is kind of weird, it doesn't feel like it's a part of my body anymore.

the **PRESCRIPTION** *for*
REFLEX SYMPATHETIC DYSTROPHY/COMPLEX REGIONAL PAIN SYNDROME

The treatment of RSD/CRPS is a little different from the treatment of other forms of neuropathic pain.

An active physical/occupational therapy program is a must. Also, repeated nerve blocks and spinal cord stimulation may provide good pain relief for a minority of patients. There are also medications that can make a big difference in reducing the pain. Psychological treatments often are key to helping many patients with RSD/CRPS.

- ✓ Active PT
- ✓ Nerve blocks
- ✓ Spinal cord stimulation
- ✓ Medications
- ✓ Psychological treatments

Symptoms of RSD/CRPS

You have RSD/CRPS, a disabling nerve pain that developed after an injury or period of immobilization. This condition has been relatively ignored and misunderstood by the medical community because it is so unusual in many respects. It was historically called Reflex Sympathetic Dystrophy (RSD), but in 1994, world experts decided to change the name to Complex Regional Pain Syndrome (CRPS). Since both terms are still used today, we will use the term RSD/CRPS.

The symptoms of RSD/CRPS can occur anywhere on the body covered by skin, but by far the condition most commonly occurs in one hand or foot. RSD/CRPS patients most often describe their pain as a deep dull ache, heaviness, freezing cold, burning, skin sensitivity, and/or with sharp jolts. Often, patients describe the pain as being in a "bucket of ice" or "deep bone pain." Patients with this condition also commonly have extremely sensitive skin to the touch (allodynia).

What make RSD/CRPS different from any other pain condition are the unusual symptoms that occur within the painful region (although not all of these need to be present in every patient):

Swelling (edema):
- Patients may describe the RSD/CRPS body part as being swollen, or may report feeling as though the area is swollen; much like the feeling you get in your lips following a Novocain injection from your dentist.

Skin color changes:
- Patients often describe the area as being deep purple, mottled, pale, red, or a blotchy color.
- Temperature changes:
- Patients say the affected side can feel cold or hot, or can change from hot to cold, as compared to the normal side.

Abnormal sweating:
- Patients may experience increased or decreased sweating on the affected side as compared to the normal side.

Changes in nails:
- Patients' nails may become very brittle or grow very long due to lack of cutting because they can be so painful to touch.

What's New: Reversible Brain Changes in RSD/CRPS

Several new scientific findings have shown abnormalities in the brain and peripheral nerves of RSD/CRPS patients. Studies performed with RSD/CRPS patients have strongly suggested that functional brain changes and skin abnormalities may be underlying some RSD/CRPS symptoms, all of which are likely reversible.

What are some of these changes? A recent study demonstrated that RSD/CRPS patients had shrinkage of their somatosensory cortex (the brain area responsible for physical sensations), which was normalized after treatment that improved their symptoms. Another important study recently found very small abnormal nerves in the skin of RSD/CRPS patients that require special laboratory testing to detect.

How can they be reversed? All of these changes in the brain, spinal cord, and also skin can likely be reversed by proper pain management and, probably more importantly, by simply using the RSD/CRPS-affected limb normally to perform daily simple tasks, such as walking, feeding oneself, or opening doors!

Weakness and motor control difficulties:
- Patients may feel as though the limb is weak.
- Patients may drop objects with hand involvement or trip with foot involvement.

Neglect:
- *Neglect* is a neurological term that describes when a patient feels as though the involved hand or leg is no longer part of his or her body, or when the patient needs to mentally focus and look at the limb to move it.
- Patients may describe the need to concentrate and look at the limb to move it.

Tremors:
- The patient may develop a mild tremor in the involved limb.

RSD/CRSP pain does not follow a pattern expected in a neurologic condition. The affected body part changes color and temperature quite dramatically, and patients often display protective behavior of their painful limb that looks odd to a doctor. Luckily, over the past several years, much new scientific evidence is demonstrating that there are real abnormalities in the nervous system and perhaps some changes in the patient's immune system that may be involved in this very disabling nerve pain condition.

TWO TYPES OF RSD/CRPS

RSD/CRPS is subdivided into two types: RSD/CRPS-Type 1 and RSD/CRPS-Type 2; to make it even more complicated, another old term sometimes used for CRPS-2 is *causalgia*. **For both types, the symptoms and treatments are exactly the same**. The only difference is that Type 1 (RSD) is caused by a musculoskeletal injury (e.g., bone, muscle, ligament, or tendon) and Type 2 (causalgia) is caused by a well-defined nerve injury. However, note that most scientists now believe that even in Type 1 there is a nerve injury, but it is too small to detect with current laboratory tests; in fact, small skin biopsies recently have found abnormal nerves in RSD/CRPS-Type 1 patients.

NO CURE, BUT SIGNIFICANT IMPROVEMENT IS POSSIBLE

The overall treatment goal is to restore normal function to the RSD/CRPS body region. Whether medication, nerve blocks, and/or spinal cord stimulators are used, the goal is to reduce the pain and symptoms, and thereby improve the patient's ability to participate in rehabilitation therapy, such as active physical and occupational therapy programs.

Although there is no definitive cure for RSD/CRPS (apart from the uncommon patients who experience complete remission if nerve blocks are done early and who maintain intensive PT), the good news is that most RSD/CRPS patients do find they can get meaningful relief and return of physical function if the condition is treated properly. **The key in RSD/CRPS is to find experienced doctors and physical/occupational therapists who have successfully taken care of many patients with RSD/CRPS.**

Diagnosing RSD/CRPS

This may be confusing due to all the name changes. What's important for you to understand now is that all pain experts now call this condition *Complex Regional Pain Syndrome* and use the CRPS diagnostic criteria to make the diagnosis. As we mentioned earlier, we are still using the RSD name in this book because some doctors who are not pain experts still mistakenly call it by this old name.

The group of experts who met in 1994 agreed to rename the condition *Complex Regional Pain Syndrome*, and after days of deliberation also agreed to a well-defined way in which to make the diagnosis (so-called diagnostic criteria). The diagnostic criteria for CRPS are strictly clinical, meaning they are based solely on information gathered from the patient's history (what the patient tells the doctor) and examination. Unlike the ways some doctors used to diagnose this condition back when it was called RSD, there is no need for nerve blocks or laboratory tests to make the diagnosis of CRPS. (The only time a laboratory test might be needed is to document a nerve injury for RSD/CRPS-Type 2.)

RSD/CRPS Alert!

Higher Risk for Psychological Disorders RSD/CRPS patients are at particular risk for developing psychological disorders, such as depression, anxiety, and PTSD, because of their severe pain and disability and also because, unfortunately, many people they deal with (doctors, insurance carriers, workers' compensation administrators) don't understand or believe their symptoms.

Who Gets RSD/CRPS?

It remains unknown why only some people develop RSD/CRPS and most do not, or why many more women than men get RSD/CRPS:

- Studies have shown that two to five times more women are afflicted than men. Studies have also reported that white women seem to be the most prevalent group with RSD/CRPS, at least in the United States.

- It also remains unknown why RSD/CRPS can develop after the fifth ankle sprain in a person while the first four sprains healed normally. No risk factors for developing RSD/CRPS have been found. It may be that everyone is at risk for developing this condition after surgery, nerve injury, or a minor trauma, such as a sprain, strain, or contusion.

- Some authorities (including us) believe that an extended time of immobilization and disuse of the involved limb following the injury may predispose some people to RSD/CRPS.

(continued)

THE DIAGNOSTIC CRITERIA FOR RSD/CRPS

- Pain and symptoms following an injury or immobilization:
  - Type 1: The pain and symptoms follow a musculoskeletal injury.
  - Type 2: The pain and symptoms follow a documented nerve injury.
  AND
- Spontaneous pain and skin sensitivity:
  - Type 1: The skin region involved does not follow a typical nerve pattern (it typically involves the entire foot or hand).
  - Type 2: The skin region involved does follow a typical nerve pattern.
  AND
- Evidence at some time of (swelling (edema), abnormal skin temperature changes (cold, hot, or both, > 1.1°C), abnormal skin color changes, and/or abnormal sudomotor activity (e.g., excessive sweating or dryness) within the region of pain.

In the past, some doctors suggested using a bone scan to help make the diagnosis, but now most authorities believe that a bone scan is not useful in diagnosis or treatment recommendations. The same goes for thermography testing—there is no need to have such a test to make the diagnosis; a skin thermometer works just fine.

EXAMINATION FINDINGS: RSD/CRPS

The painful body part in RSD/CRPS is most often located in a limb on only one side of the body. Compared to the uninvolved limb on the other side, the RSD/CRPS area may be swollen; be abnormal in color (blotchy, red, or purple); be abnormal in temperature (hot and/or cold); and sweat profusely, often quite suddenly, or alternatively, never sweat at all. **Because the examination findings in RSD/CRPS can change minute by minute, it is important that the examining doctor evaluates the patient during more than one appointment.**

Also quite often, when RSD/CRPS occurs in the arm or hand the patient holds the upper extremity tightly against his or her body, in a guarded position. This guarding behavior classically was thought to be due to the patient's conscious decision to protect his or her RSD/CRPS limb from someone touching it, which would cause a worsening of pain. However, several reports have strongly suggested that in some RSD/CRPS patients, this guarding may happen involuntarily, due to dysfunction in a certain part of the brain. (Note that this is not injury to the brain, but rather is likely a reversible chemical imbalance in the brain, with the exact chemical not yet known at the time of this writing).

In addition to having some weakness in the RSD/CRPS limb, many RSD/CRPS patients have difficulty initiating or making their RSD/CRPS limb move. These patients may tell their doctor that to move the involved hand/arm or foot/leg, they need to concentrate on the limb and look at it. This symptom can be verified on examination and is called *motor neglect*. The cause is not known.

On sensory examination, some abnormalities may be observed in the RSD/CRPS area. These sensory changes may include numbness or loss of sensation to light touch, cold, and pinprick. However, the patient may describe other regions as being abnormally sensitive to light touch (allodynia). Importantly, these sensory changes in RSD/CRPS-Type 1 do not follow a typical peripheral nerve distribution. They usually involve the entire foot or hand. The reason for this pattern of involvement is not known, but it is thought to be due to changes in the spinal cord or brain.

RSD/CRPS Explained (Or Not)

The underlying cause of RSD/CRPS remains unknown, though there is a tremendous amount of research now being performed to better understand RSD/CRPS.

By definition, the development of RSD/CRPS follows a musculoskeletal injury, nerve injury, or immobilization (not moving the limb). However, usually the injury is very minor, such as a sprain, strain, contusion, or even a stub of the toe.

Currently, most pain authorities believe abnormal changes in both the peripheral and central nervous systems cause this disorder. This has been demonstrated in studies over the past several years. Some experts believe that something abnormal happens during the body's natural healing reaction to injury. Natural responses to a local injury include an inflammatory response that causes the area to become red, warm, and swollen. Such normal changes are accompanied by changes in the nervous system, which alter the pain sensations in the surrounding areas, resulting in increased skin sensitivity and tenderness.

We've all experienced these normal, natural changes with a contusion or joint sprain, all of which diminish and resolve over a short period of time. But in RSD/CRPS, they may continue indefinitely and actually become exaggerated. One hypothesis is that RSD/CRPS represents a disruption of the normal healing process, although it is not known how the pain and other RSD/CRPS symptoms are maintained over months and even years.

(Who Gets RSD/CRPS? continued)

- Though it's not proven, we also believe that experiencing an increased amount of stress at the time of an injury may make development of RSD/CRPS more likely.

- There is no proof of a genetic predisposition to developing this disorder, although here, too, some experts think this may play a role, at least in some patients.

- It has been definitively shown that there is no psychological predisposition to developing RSD/CRPS.

89

Get the Facts: Dispelling Myths about RSD/CRPS

The following are true statements based on scientific fact:

- RSD/CRPS is not caused by psychological disturbance.
- There are no definite "stages" that patients with RSD/CRPS go through.
- Most patients' RSD/CRPS symptoms do not spread.
- Most patients do not respond to sympathetic nerve blocks.

The Natural Course of RSD/CRPS

The true natural history and expected course for this disorder is not known. However, unlike what some Web sites incorrectly state, **RSD/CRPS does not and should not result in amputation or the patient becoming wheelchair-bound.** Studies that evaluate what happens to RSD/CRPS patients over time show that some symptoms resolve with proper treatment, but many unfortunately remain chronic. So much depends on whether the patient receives the proper treatment.

Most authorities agree, however, that if a patient stops moving the RSD/CRPS limb and does not use it as he or she normally would, the symptoms will not improve. Also, further complications can develop when the RSD/CRPS limb is not used, including tight muscles, tendons, and ligaments in areas adjacent to the RSD/CRPS region.

Does RSD/CRPS spread? Many patients describe a spreading of pain and symptoms. However, in the experience of most pain doctors (us included), the spreading of pain and symptoms in RSD/CRPS is most often not due to an actual spreading of the RSD/CRPS, but rather to myofascial dysfunction in muscles, tendons, and ligaments that are not being used properly. For instance, if you have RSD/CRPS in your hand, you likely are not using that hand and arm as you normally would. You then start to develop tight and spastic muscles in your shoulder and neck, resulting in pain in those regions, and also probably a tension-type headache. If you have RSD/CRPS in your foot, you likely will develop tight and spastic muscles in your hip, buttocks, and lower back, with pain developing in those regions as well.

CONCLUSION: NEUROPATHIC PAIN IS EASILY DIAGNOSED AND TREATED

If you have a neuropathic pain condition, you are actually quite lucky to be living today. So much has been learned over the past decade about nerve pain, and we have seen a huge increase in the number of medications and treatments that can safely help people suffering from all types of neuropathic pain. So, be optimistic. The diagnoses of most neuropathic pain conditions are easy to make; lots of safe treatment options are available; and many pharmaceutical companies are developing even more medications to treat your type of pain.

What is a typical drug regimen for a patient with PHN pain?

We need to reiterate that every patient should be on the least amount of medication that provides the best balance of good pain relief and few if any side effects. However, many PHN (and other neuropathic pain) patients may need several drugs. We always try a topical drug first, usually the lidocaine patch 5% (Lidoderm). If that gives some good relief but the patient is still suffering from moderate pain, we'll add one oral medication, either gabapentin (Neurontin), pregabalin (Lyrica), or duloxetine (Cymbalta).

I just saw a TV show about mirror therapy. Can this help with RSD/CRPS?

Yes! This new type of treatment is exciting and has been shown in studies to help with some of the symptoms of RSD/CRPS (and also with phantom limb pain). With mirror therapy, the patient simply looks into a mirror while he or she is moving his or her healthy unaffected limb; this tricks the brain into thinking it is the painful limb that is moving. It's quite cool, and it works!

My doctor has tried all types of medication for my diabetic neuropathy pain—all of the non-narcotics you mention. But he will not prescribe an opioid narcotic to me, as he says it won't work and can cause addiction. What should I do?

Your dilemma is unfortunately common. First, we recommend you bring him this book to show him that good clinical studies have shown that opioid narcotics can significantly relieve neuropathic pain and that in treating pain in a patient without a history of addiction the risk of creating an addiction is extremely low. If your doctor is still reluctant, we suggest you be evaluated by an experienced pain doctor (hopefully with your current doctor's blessing).

CHAPTER 5

Obliterating Headaches
(Migraine/Tension-Type/Rebound)

Not all headaches are created equal—

proper diagnosis is critical for pain relief.

the PRESCRIPTION for MIGRAINE HEADACHE

If you have fewer than three headaches per month, try taking an over-the-counter (OTC) analgesic, such as acetaminophen (Tylenol), ibuprofen (Motrin, Advil), or naproxen (Aleve), at the start of the headache.

If those don't work, you can take a prescription headache medication when you get a headache, or if you have frequent debilitating headaches every month you can take a medication every day to prevent headaches. Nonmedication therapies such as yoga and biofeedback also show good results in relieving migraines.

- ✓ OTC drugs
- ✓ Prescription medications to treat headache
- ✓ Prescription medications to prevent headaches
- ✓ Yoga
- ✓ Trigger-point injections (TPIs)
- ✓ Biofeedback
- ✓ Stress reduction

Migraine Headache:
A Patient's Story

I'm a 23-year-old woman. I've had headaches ever since I was a teenager, coinciding with my first menstrual period. I've had them nearly every month since then. Although my symptoms have never varied much, they are beginning to interfere with my life, and now the headaches appear to be unrelated to my menstrual cycle. I have one-sided throbbing pain over my temple and forehead, usually on the right side. Within 15 to 30 minutes, it becomes very severe, a 10/10 pain, and the other symptoms develop, including nausea, vomiting, and sensitivity to light and sound. These are just ruining my life.

Menstrual Migraine

About 60 percent of women who have migraines experience an increase in association with their menstrual period. In 10 percent to 14 percent of these women, migraines occur only around the time of their period. Migraines that increase in frequency or severity around the time of the menstrual period are referred to as *menstrual migraines*. Most headache specialists conclude that a patient is suffering from a menstrual migraine if 90 percent of her migraines occur between the two days before and the last day of her menstrual period.

Studies have shown that menstrual migraines are usually more resistant to treatment, are more severe, last longer, and may be associated with greater disability, as compared to other migraines. Still, specific medications can be quite effective in treating this disorder.

Although the other theories for general migraines can also be applied to menstrual migraines, the characteristic trigger for menstrual migraines, menstruation, strongly suggests a hormonal basis for this migraine type. Many studies, both biochemical and genetic, strongly suggest the rapid changes in estrogen levels as the major trigger for menstrual migraines.

Migraine, Tension-Type, and Rebound Headaches

Headaches are one of the most common medical problems, and often can be resolved with OTC pain relievers. However, for hundreds of millions of people around the world, headaches can be severe and even disabling, rendering them bed-bound or causing major disruptions in their lives. Believe it or not, more than 150 different types of headaches have been described in the medical literature, each with its own set of symptoms and treatments. In this chapter, we will focus on the three most common types: migraine, tension-type, and rebound headaches.

Symptoms of a Migraine Headache

You have a migraine headache—a throbbing pain over one side of your forehead or temple. Sometimes before the migraine, you may see flashing zigzag lines, letting you know a big one is coming. Within fifteen to thirty minutes, your pain becomes very severe and other symptoms—such as nausea, vomiting, and sensitivity to light—set in. Once the headache quiets down (which can take many hours), you probably feel exhausted and just want to sleep in a dark, quiet room.

Despite what many people think, a migraine isn't just a severe pain in the head. To be classified as a migraine, the pain has to be accompanied by other symptoms, such as gastrointestinal distress or sensitivity to light and sound. Some patients with migraines experience aura, which are sensory symptoms that occur before the migraine pain begins. The most common symptom is visual, usually described as flashing lights or zigzag lines. Other patients with aura may experience unusual smells, though this is not common.

Medications To Manage Migraines

The many medications available for managing migraine can be broken down into two broad classes: acute migraine medications and chronic migraine medications (or preventive migraine medications). Acute medications are used to treat the migraine while it is happening—the patient takes the drug once he or she starts to experience symptoms. Chronic medications are taken every day by patients who regularly experience migraines, with the goal of preventing or reducing the number of attacks.

Acute Migraine Medications
TRIPTANS SPELL RELIEF FROM MIGRAINES

Triptan medications are considered the best prescription medications for the acute treatment of migraines. Many different triptans are currently prescribed in the United States, including sumatriptan (Imitrex), frovatriptan (Frova), zolmitriptan (Zomig), eletriptan (Relpax), naratriptan (Amerge), and rizatriptan (Maxalt). These medications work by interacting with specific neurotransmitter receptors in the brain or scalp—namely the serotonin 1B and 1D receptors—and thereby cause a reduction in the brain chemical inflammation associated with migraines. All of the triptans have been shown to quickly relieve the pain of migraines, as well as reduce and sometimes eliminate nausea, vomiting, and light or noise sensitivity associated with the condition.

Migraine Alert!

Changes in Pregnancy and Menopause Some pregnancies cause a worsening of migraines and others result in some improvement of the condition. After menopause, migraines typically either reduces significantly or completely resolves. Although there is definitely a link between migraines and female hormones, the exact mechanism is still not known. It is believed that the brain areas that cause migraines may be more sensitive to changing hormone levels in some women that occur each month and throughout a woman's life.

When Taking Medications: Every person with migraines is different and will react differently to medication.

It is better to take acute medication as soon as you realize you are about to have a migraine. If you take a drug after the full-blown migraine has already happened, it is less likely that you will experience significant pain relief.

Taking too much of any acute migraine drug will result in a worse headache condition called rebound headache syndrome. Headache experts recommend that a patient take no more than ten doses of acute migraine medication per month.

Migraine Alert!

Improper Use of OTC NSAID Medications Can Lead To:

- Immediate stomach irritation
- Serious or fatal kidney and liver toxicity (when taken too frequently or for too long)
- Rebound headache syndrome (discussed later in this chapter)
- Heart problems if taken chronically (classic NSAIDs)

ACUTE MIGRAINE DRUGS AVAILABLE OTC

Most migraine patients are able to treat their headaches with nonprescription, OTC painkillers such as acetaminophen (Tylenol), aspirin, classic nonsteroidal anti-inflammatory drugs or NSAIDs (Aleve, Motrin, Advil), or the combination of acetaminophen, aspirin, and caffeine (Excedrin). All of these drugs are in your local drugstore's analgesic aisle. Analgesic means "pain reliever." They all have serious potential side effects (see "Migraine Alert!").

These medications work by reducing the action of COX enzymes and prostaglandins—agents thought to be responsible for the pain and inflammation associated with migraines. All NSAIDs have been shown to be effective for some people with migraines, though usually not as effective as triptans.

CLASSIC NSAIDS AND COX-2 INHIBITOR DRUGS

Some patients with migraines need prescription-strength classic NSAIDs for adequate relief. Other patients select COX-2 inhibitors, such as Celebrex, a newer class of NSAID medication which offers pain relief with a reduced risk for some of the acute gastrointestinal symptoms associated with classic NSAIDs. However, all prescription NSAIDs have the potential to cause stomach irritation and are associated with the same side effects as the OTC NSAIDs (as we discussed earlier).

UNDESIRABLE PRESCRIPTION ACUTE MIGRAINE MEDICATIONS

For several decades, especially before triptans were discovered, several other medications were prescribed for the treatment of migraines: barbiturates, ergotamines, antinausea medications, and short-acting opioids. Although all of these drugs have been shown to help alleviate the pain (or other symptoms) of migraines in certain patients, the drugs for various reasons are not currently first-line medications.

Chronic Migraine Medications (Preventive Migraine Medication)

Chronic migraine medications are taken every day, even when the patient is not experiencing pain. The goal of this therapy is to reduce the number and severity of migraines over time. Most headache specialists prescribe preventive migraine medication only to patients who have at least two or more migraine attacks per month or experience at least four days per month when their ability to perform their daily activities is severely affected. Additionally, many doctors will prescribe preventive migraine medication only after multiple acute migraine drugs have been tried without success. Currently, the FDA has approved four preventive medications for migraine.

PROPRANOLOL AND TIMOLOL ARE BETA BLOCKERS

Propranolol (Inderal) and timolol (Blocadren) are primarily used in the treatment of high blood pressure and heart disease. Common side effects include fatigue, cold hands, weakness, and dizziness.

VALPROIC ACID AND TOPIRAMATE STABILIZE NERVES

Originally developed for the management of epilepsy, valproic acid (Depakote) and topiramate (Topamax) are thought to prevent migraine by stabilizing abnormal nerve activity in the brain. Both of these drugs can be very effective in preventing migraine attacks. However, they can also lead to potentially serious side effects. Valproic acid has more possible side effects than topiramate, such as significant weight gain and liver toxicity in some patients. Overall, topiramate is better tolerated than valproic acid, but both drugs can cause sedation and trouble thinking and, rarely, serious skin reactions.

Triptan Alert!

Not for the Faint of Heart
Before taking any triptan, your doctor should evaluate your risk factors for heart disease: high blood pressure, high cholesterol, diabetes, a history of smoking, Raynaud's disease, a history of stroke or TIAs ("mini strokes"), and peripheral vascular disease. **If you have any of these risk factors, you should not be prescribed any triptan drug. All triptan medications have been associated with a very small but real increased risk of heart attack in patients with these risk factors.**

If One Triptan Doesn't Work, Try Another

Each triptan drug works a little differently on the serotonin chemicals in the brain. Some studies have shown that a patient may do well with one triptan and not another. Therefore, it may be worthwhile to try at least two of these drugs before giving up on triptans.

The most common side effects from triptans are:
• A sense of bodily warmth
• Chest tightness and palpitations
• Dizziness
• Tingling sensations
• The potential for heart attack or stroke

Nondrug Therapies For Migraine

In addition to the many medications available for the treatment of migraines, some patients benefit from nondrug therapies. In particular, these types of therapies seem to work best in patients who find tight and tender muscles in their head and neck during and before migraines, and some help migraine sufferers who find that their headaches occur more often during stressful times in their life.

HEADACHE/PAIN CLINICS PROVIDE COMPREHENSIVE CARE

Most often, migraine pain can be successfully managed by a primary care physician. However, if you suffer from frequent, debilitating migraines that cannot be resolved in this setting, you can still find excellent relief with a headache specialist or in a comprehensive headache/pain clinic. These clinics have the tools needed to treat migraine in a holistic manner, with such therapies as medication management, physical therapy (PT), biofeedback, stress management, and sometimes acupuncture.

TRIGGER-POINT INJECTIONS REDUCE MUSCLE SPASMS

As we described in chapter 1, TPIs are aimed at reducing the focal spasm of the muscles that are causing pain. For migraines, TPIs should be used only if you have well-defined trigger points in your shoulders, neck, and/or head muscles. A variety of different techniques for TPIs can be used (see chapter 9). All of these methods are supported by evidence suggesting that they can relieve myofascial pain for days, weeks, or months.

NERVE BLOCKS CAN NUMB THE MIGRAINE PAIN

For many years, prior to the discovery of acute migraine drugs such as triptans, some doctors performed greater occipital nerve blocks to treat migraine attacks. To perform this fairly simple nerve block, a doctor injects a medication such as Novocain into the greater occipital nerve, which lies very close to the skin on the back of the head. This specific type of nerve block continues to be used frequently in some countries in Asia.

HEAT WRAPS FOR TIGHT, TENDER MUSCLES

Although typically not well studied in patients with migraines, some migraine sufferers who get tight and tender muscles in their neck and shoulders (myofascial dysfunction) may find that OTC heat wraps (e.g., ThermaCare) can possibly reduce their migraines.

STRESS MANAGEMENT CALMS THE TRIGGER

Stress has been demonstrated to be a common trigger for many migraine patients; therefore, tools that reduce the body's reaction to stress will often decrease the frequency, intensity, and duration of migraine attacks. Stress has a direct effect on muscle tension and brain chemistry, both of which are thought to play an important role in migraines. Thus, learning stress management techniques, such as relaxation training and therapeutic imagery, can reduce the frequency and intensity of migraines.

Trigger-Point Alert!

Injections Can Be Painful
Be aware that the first few injections can be quite painful. The injected muscle may actually go into a deeper spasm before it eventually relaxes.

Table 5.1: Additional Nondrug Strategies for the Management of Migraines	
Acupuncture	• Studies have shown mixed results when evaluating acupuncture for migraines. Some studies have shown good results, while other studies have reported results similar to placebo-acupuncture.
Biofeedback	• Many studies have demonstrated very good results from biofeedback as both an acute and a preventive treatment for migraines. • Patients should look for a biofeedback provider with specific training in treating headaches
Massage/ acupressure/ craniosacral manipulation	• Many patients with migraines, especially those with myofascial dysfunction, find that regular massage, acupressure, or craniosacral manipulation treatments can help with the frequency and severity of migraines.
Rehabilitation/PT	• Studies have shown that aerobic conditioning (an exercise program) with neck and shoulder exercises that reduce tension in these muscles can be of benefit to patients with migraines. • The key is to find a health care provider who is trained specifically to treat headaches.

What's New: Heat Treatments and Yoga for Migraines

One type of heat treatment that some doctors are currently using for migraines is focal heat trigger-point (FHTP) therapy. This technique seems to work only for migraine sufferers who also find tight, tender muscle knots in their neck and shoulders during and between migraines. This therapy uses a focused, controlled heat source applied directly to the myofascial trigger point, similar to a TPI but without the need for a doctor to do it. Zeno is one device that some patients find helpful. It is approved by the FDA to treat acne, and provides a focused area of time-limited and safe heat.

Yoga helps with migraines

Although the treatment itself is ancient, recent studies have found that practicing yoga can help alleviate migraines. One study compared yoga, which included gentle yoga postures, breathing practices, relaxation, and meditation, to "normal" treatment that included diet and lifestyle changes. The researchers found that patients who did yoga therapy one hour each day for three months reported a reduction in the frequency and intensity of their migraine attacks, whereas the other patients experienced no change or worsened.

As we describe more fully in chapter 17, you can "calm" your nervous system and body to minimize your reaction to stress in many different ways. Some of the more common techniques include meditation, music- or sound-induced relaxation, mental imagery, and rhythmic, deep, visualized, or diaphragmatic breathing. Many patients find relaxation CDs, tapes, and videos to be very helpful. Don't give up if the first one you try doesn't seem to work. Try several, as you may respond better to one method or even to a person's voice (you won't get a good relaxation response if a voice reminds you of an ex-boyfriend or girlfriend!).

Your Favorite Place

One technique that works for many folks is therapeutic imagery, which allows you to "escape to your favorite place." If you can bring your thoughts and imagination to your favorite peaceful place, whether it's lying on a sunny beach or unwinding next to a roaring fire, your body and mind will begin to relax and melt away your stress reaction.

Patients can acquire these stress management skills by seeking a cognitive behavioral therapist (usually a psychologist) specializing in headache/pain management, or by visiting a pain clinic. Additional nonmedication therapies recommended for the management of migraine are outlined in Table 5.1.

YOU DON'T HAVE TO GIVE UP ALL YOUR FAVORITE FOODS!

Although some migraine sufferers should avoid certain types of food, these restrictions should be taken with a grain of salt because every migraine patient is different. No one food or beverage will uniformly cause a migraine in every patient. Therefore, a "one-size-fits-all" migraine diet is overly simplistic. To instruct all migraine patients not to consume alcohol, chocolate, coffee, or foods that contain tyramine (e.g., aged cheese, beer, and red wine) is just silly and just plain wrong.

Of course, certain foods can and will provoke a migraine in some patients. People with migraine should find out which foods are their poisons. If a patient is not aware of which foods may trigger his or her migraine, the individual should keep a food diary for one month and try to find out which foods and beverages, if any, will bring on an attack, and then try to avoid those specific

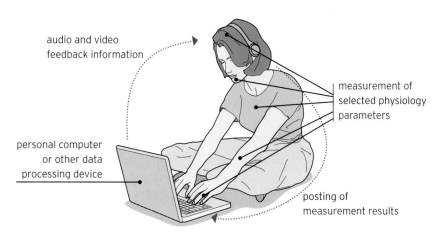

audio and video
feedback information

measurement of
selected physiology
parameters

personal computer
or other data
processing device

posting of
measurement results

The Promise of Biofeedback

Biofeedback has been used successfully for decades to help many patients with migraines. In fact, it has become one of the more frequently recommended nonmedication therapies by headache specialists. Simply put, biofeedback is another way to teach you how to control your body's stress reaction by helping you to learn how to control certain bodily functions, such as blood pressure, heart rate, skin temperature, sweat gland activity, and muscle tension. With biofeedback, you are hooked up to a biofeedback machine by simple sensors attached to your skin. These sensors allow you to obtain information regarding your bodily functions in real time, either by showing waves on a computer screen or by playing different pitches of noise. A trained biofeedback therapist will teach you how to become aware of these internal bodily functions and how to control them. The eventual goal of biofeedback is for you to be able to recognize and control your stress reactions, even without the biofeedback machine.

items in the future. Some of the more common (but by no means universal) migraine dietary triggers are red wine, chocolate, nuts, processed meats, and MSG. Interestingly, coffee is a migraine trigger for some people, while for others it actually relieves migraine.

WHEN SLEEP IS PART OF THE PROBLEM

Studies have shown that improving your sleep can have a significant positive effect on your migraines. Many people around the world do not have a proper night's sleep. However, by following these simple steps, most folks can improve their sleep every night:

- Don't go to bed watching *Dexter*! And for that matter, don't go to sleep watching any television or doing email in bed. Shut off all electronics.
- Reduce your caffeine intake, especially after lunchtime. (We Starbucks junkies know how hard it is to do this!)
- Exercise, exercise, exercise! But do it in the morning, not in the evening.
- Don't eat anything substantial for several hours prior to bedtime.
- Eat dinner at least three hours before you get in bed. Some experts recommend a snack high in carbohydrates such as cereal and milk, or a bagel, which may induce sleep by boosting levels of serotonin.

101

Surgery Is Not an Option
There is no role for surgery in the treatment for migraine headaches. In particular, removing female organs (the ovaries and uterus) is not a treatment for menstrual migraines!

Diagnosing Migraines

The diagnosis of migraines is purely clinical, based only on how the person describes his or her headache. For a person to be diagnosed with migraines, his or her neurological examination and laboratory tests must be completely normal. No currently available tests can identify a patient who has the condition. Some patients with migraines might have tight and tender head, neck, and shoulder muscles, which is referred to as *myofascial dysfunction*. During a migraine attack, many patients find that their head and scalp are painfully sensitive to light touching or stroking. The presently accepted diagnostic criteria for migraines come from the International Headache Society (IHS) and are described inTable 5.2.

Migraines Explained

The occurrence of migraines in a given individual depends on both predisposing and precipitating factors. The primary predisposing factor in patients with migraines is their genetic makeup, or family history of the condition. However, many environmental factors—such as hormonal changes, food intake, sleep patterns, and stress level—often affect the frequency and severity of these headaches. These precipitating environmental factors can all trigger migraines.

Table 5.2: Diagnostic Criteria for Migraines

Patients with migraines report at least five attacks, with each attack lasting four to seventy-two hours untreated or unsuccessfully treated, and meeting the following criteria:

Headaches have at least two of these characteristics:	• Unilateral (one-sided) • Pulsating or throbbing quality • Moderate or severe intensity (inhibits or prohibits daily activities) • Worsening when walking up stairs or performing similar physical activity
During the headache, at least one of these occurs:	• Nausea and/or vomiting • Photophobia (sensitivity to light) and phonophobia (sensitivity to sound)

ABNORMAL BRAIN PROCESSES IN MIGRAINES

For many years, doctors and researchers have discussed multiple theories of migraine. Each theory is supported by some evidence, but none appear to be able to completely explain the entire set of symptoms found in this condition. Some of today's most popular theories used to explain how a migraine occurs in the brain are outlined in Table 5.3.

Table 5.3: Theories about Migraines	
The vascular theory (disproved!)	Migraines have two stages: • Stage 1: The brain's blood vessels constrict • Stage 2: The brain's blood vessels dilate, causing throbbing pain
The spreading depression theory	• Migraines are caused by a slow-moving energy field that starts in the back of the brain and moves forward to trigger migraines
The serotonergic theory	• Migraines are caused by changes in the amount of the neurochemical serotonin in particular parts of the brain
The neurovascular theory	• Migraines are caused by inflammation of the trigeminovascular system, a specific area of the brain thought to be responsible for several kinds of headaches
The meningeal inflammatory theory	• Migraines are caused by inflammation of the meninges, the thin, skin-like covering of the brain
The mixed theory (what we believe)	• Abnormalities in blood vessels, neurotransmitters, meninges, and other factors work together to cause migraines. In some patients one of these factors may contribute more than others, but all can play a part in the development of a migraine

Tension Type Headache History:
A Patient's Story

I'm a 23-year-old man and had never experienced headaches until a year ago, when I got a promotion and more responsibility with my job. And now the headaches are occurring more frequently, about one bad headache per week. The pain starts at the base of my neck and then moves to my entire head, like a belt tightening around my head. Occasionally I have other symptoms—about a third of the time I have some mild nausea and sensitivity to light. Now the headaches also cause my neck to feel stiff and sore. I have not seen any doctors about this problem, but have been self-medicating with over-the-counter preparations, such as acetaminophen, ibuprofen, and aspirin. They are really not helping. What can I do?

the PRESCRIPTION for TENSION-TYPE HEADACHES

Although tension-type headaches are more common than migraines, few treatments for this condition have been well studied.

And believe it or not, no acute or preventive treatment has obtained FDA approval to treat tension-type headaches. Nevertheless, many therapies, both medication and nonmedication treatments, can be effective in alleviating the pain of tension-type headache.

- ✓ Acute medication
- ✓ Preventive medication
- ✓ Acupuncture
- ✓ Biofeedback
- ✓ Heat
- ✓ TPI
- ✓ Stress reduction

Symptoms of Tension-Type Headaches

You have a tension-type headache, with pain that starts in your neck and then moves into your head. It feels like a belt tightening around your head and is accompanied by stiffness or soreness in the neck. You may find some relief from taking OTC pain medications, and sometimes a hot shower helps. There is no nausea and very little, if any, light sensitivity.

A tension-type headache occurs on both sides of the head and is described as pressing or tightening pain—people often liken it to a vise or a tight belt around the head. Thus, a tension-type headache is different from a migraine, which is one-sided and is felt as a pulsating or throbbing pain. There is no nausea, but some people with tension-type headaches may experience sensitivity to either light or sound (but not both), or will complain of feeling dizzy or lightheaded. Many patients with tension-type headaches also experience tight, tender neck and head muscles (myofascial dysfunction).

The most common form of tension-type headaches is the episodic type, meaning that headaches come and go, whereas the more disabling chronic type occurs nearly every day. Luckily, chronic tension-type headaches occur in fewer than 5 percent of the population.

Acute Tension-Type Headache Medication

The drugs we discuss in this section are designed to be taken either at the onset or during a tension-type headache in the hope of alleviating headache pain (and, in some cases, myofascial pain).

Tension-Type Alert!

What's in a Name?
Tension-type may be a misleading name for this disorder, as it may imply that these headaches are purely psychological or stress-related, which is not the case. Prior to 1988, this headache condition was called muscle-contraction headache, which might be a more appropriate name for most cases of this condition.

105

OTC ACUTE TENSION-TYPE HEADACHE DRUGS
The most commonly used drugs to treat tension-type headaches are nonprescription OTC analgesics. As we described in the OTC Migraine Headache Drugs section (the medications are the same), all of these drugs can lead to acute and long-term adverse reactions.

PRESCRIPTION ACUTE TENSION-TYPE HEADACHE MEDICATIONS
Some patients with tension-type headaches find that they need prescription-strength classic NSAID drugs or COX-2 inhibitors to treat their pain.

PREVENTIVE TENSION-TYPE HEADACHE MEDICATION
Preventive tension-type headache medications are taken every day (regardless of whether a headache is present that day) in the hopes of preventing or reducing the number of attacks in the future. Although no drug is currently FDA-approved for the prevention of tension-type headaches, several drugs can offer some patients relief. Headache specialists sometimes prescribe the following drugs as preventive medication to chronic tension-type headache patients: tricyclic antidepressants (TCAs), gabapentin, and topiramate.

Nondrug Therapies For Tension-Type Headaches
Many nondrug therapies are available for management of tension-type headaches, as listed in Table 5.4.

Diagnosing Tension-Type Headache
As in patients with migraines, the results of the neurological examination and laboratory tests of a patient with tension-type headaches are completely normal. The only abnormality seen on examination of tension-type headache patients is that they often have very tight and tender muscles and myofascial trigger points in their neck, shoulders, and/or head. They also may have poor range of motion in these areas. As with migraines, the diagnosis of tension-type headaches is solely based on clinical criteria, which have been written by the International Headache Society (IHS).

Table 5.4: Therapies for Management of Tension-Type Headaches

Acupuncture	This ancient Chinese treatment has been shown in several good scientific studies to be of benefit, either alone or in combination with medication to treat tension-type headaches
Biofeedback	By learning to control certain body reactions to stress, including muscle tension in the neck, shoulders, and head, biofeedback can result in a significant reduction in pain severity and the frequency of tension-type headaches
Headache/pain clinic	A specialized headache or pain clinic can provide a thorough evaluation of your headache problem and then tailor a specific treatment regimen for your tension-type headache condition, including both medication and nonmedication therapies
Heat treatment/massage	If your tension-type headache has a large underlying component of muscle tension in your neck, shoulders, and head, applying heat to these muscles and/or getting a focused massage may be of therapeutic benefit
Rehabilitation/PT	Quite often, patients with tension-type headaches who have an underlying muscle problem in their neck and shoulders may have an underlying posture or chronic myofascial dysfunction problem that will need a more dedicated PT program
Stress management techniques	For most patients with tension-type headaches, stress is an important trigger; therefore, learning simple stress management techniques can greatly improve the condition
Trigger Point Injections	For tension-type headache patients in which myofascial dysfunction in the neck and shoulders is involved, focused TPIs can be an important part of the treatment plan

Potential Mechanisms Underlying Tension-Type Headaches

Although there is no consensus as to the mechanisms underlying this type of headache, the three most likely theories are:

Myofascial dysfunction in the shoulders, neck, and head

Neurochemical abnormalities such as serotonin in the brain and/or nitric oxide in the muscles that may be involved in the transformation of acute into chronic tension-type headaches

A combination of 1 and 2, the amount of each depending on the individual

IHS CRITERIA FOR TENSION-TYPE HEADACHES

Patients with tension-type headaches report the following symptoms:

- Headache attacks last from thirty minutes to seven days (untreated or unsuccessfully treated).
- At least two of the following can be used to describe the headache:
  - Pain occurs on both sides of the head.
  - Pain has a pressing/tightening quality (like a vise squeezing the head).
  - Pain is of mild or moderate intensity (may inhibit but does not prohibit activities).
  - Pain is not worsened by walking, stairs, or performing similar routine physical activity.
- During the headache, both of the following apply:
  - No nausea or vomiting is present.
  - Either photophobia (sensitivity to light) or phonophobia (sensitivity to sound) may be present, but not both.

Subtypes:

Episodic tension-type headaches: Headaches occur for one or more days and fewer than fifteen days per month.

Chronic tension-type headaches: Headaches occur for fifteen or more days per month for more than three months.

Tension-Type Headaches Explained

The cause of tension-type headaches is controversial. As we mentioned earlier, this syndrome was once termed *muscle contraction headache*, since most experts believed the cause was a disorder of the muscles in the head and neck. However, in 1988, when the IHS concluded that this condition was distinct from migraine, there was much disagreement as to its cause. To reach a consensus, the experts renamed this headache subtype *tension-type headache* because they (falsely) believed this new name didn't imply any specific underlying bodily mechanism.

Myofascial dysfunction likely causes the report that many patients feel dizzy and lightheaded. Shoulder and neck muscles have a role in helping us keep our body in balance and telling our brain the location of our head. Thus, when they go into spasm, they can give the brain misinformation and cause a feeling of dizziness.

the PRESCRIPTION for REBOUND HEADACHES

The most important action patients can take to treat rebound headache syndrome is to stop taking all of their acute pain medication.

If these medications are not stopped, no additional treatments will have any effect. Studies have shown that prescribing preventive migraine medication will not have a beneficial effect if the patient continues to take his or her acute pain medication(s). For most patients with rebound headache, stress management is a crucial part of the treatment plan. Also, some patients can find some relief with biofeedback, acupuncture, and heat wrap, but all these are not crucial to the treatment plan.

- ✓ Stress management
- ✓ Biofeedback
- ✓ Acupuncture
- ✓ Heat wraps

Rebound Headache:
A Patient's Story

I've had headaches off and on since I was a teenager, but up until last year, I only experienced bad ones during my period when I was also tired and burnt-out from work or partying too hard. At the time around my divorce, about one year ago, I began to have more and more of my typical one-sided headaches, with nausea and light sensitivity. However, over the past six months, it's these new headaches that are really bothering me—every single day I get a nagging, constant pain throughout my entire head, but without nausea or sensitivity to light. I now also have neck pain. My doctor say's it's stress. I've taken everything for this: acetaminophen, ibuprofen, aspirin, naproxen. And all of them have become less and less effective, so now I've increased the dosages from one tablet a day to two or three per day. I really don't want to just keep increasing the drugs I am taking, but what else can I do?

Get the Facts: Rebound Headache Syndrome

- From 40 percent to 70 percent of patients seeking care at headache clinics may be suffering from rebound headache syndrome.

- One study reported that approximately 20 percent of patients seeking help from their primary care physician for headaches were taking excessive acute headache medications, and thus were at risk for developing this condition.

- One authority has projected that up to 1 percent of the entire population of industrialized countries may be suffering from rebound headache syndrome.

Symptoms Of Rebound Headache Syndrome

You have rebound headache syndrome. You used to get headaches once or twice per month and took acute pain medication to treat them, which always worked. However, recently these headaches have become more severe and frequent, with pain in the left temple, accompanied by nausea and light sensitivity. To make matters worse, over the past six months you have developed a new type of headache that occurs almost every day, with some neck pain. This headache feels like a nagging, constant pain, but without the nausea and light sensitivity. You have become so paranoid about getting a bad headache that you don't leave home without your pain medication (Tylenol, Motrin/Advil, Aleve, triptan, Percocet, Vicodin, etc.), even though these pills seem to be working less and less effectively.

In a classic example of rebound headache syndrome, a patient with a prior history of migraines (or episodic tension-type headaches) develops daily or near-daily headaches. Usually, but not always, the individual has some underlying trigger (most often a stressful life event) that causes him or her to have frequent headaches. Over time, after taking more and more of his or her acute headache pain medication, the individual develops a new type of headache, which is different from the original headache. These new rebound headaches occur on both sides of the head, and are described as a pressing feeling or "tight band" around the head that typically isn't as severe as the patient's old headaches but is there almost all the time. Importantly, most of these patients may also continue to have their migraine (or tension-type) headaches in addition to these new daily rebound headaches.

These new headaches have no or very little nausea and vomiting, and little light or sound sensitivity. Many patients with rebound headache syndrome also complain of feeling dizzy and lightheaded. As is the case in tension-type headaches, this symptom is likely due to myofascial dysfunction.

CHARACTERIZED BY PILL CONSUMPTION

Beyond the physical symptoms, another characteristic of rebound headache syndrome is patients' consumption of daily or near-daily acute headache pain medications. Patients typically notice that over time, their acute medication works less well and they need to take increased dosages to have the same effect (because they've developed tolerance to the medication).

Rebound headache syndrome is a severe disabling condition that can severely impede the lives of its sufferers. By the time patients develop rebound headache syndrome, it becomes a complicated condition to treat. Still, it should be noted that this syndrome is both preventable and curable! It is our goal that, by writing this book, at least one case of rebound headache syndrome may be prevented and that other individuals will realize they have the condition and receive information they need to be cured.

Table 5.5: Acute Pain Medications That Should Be Discontinued in Patients with Rebound Headache Syndrome

MEDICATION CLASS	EXAMPLES			
OTC analgesics	• Acetaminophen	• Ibuprofen	• Aspirin	• Naproxen
Prescription NSAIDs	• Ibuprofen	• Ketorolac	• Diclofenac sodium	• Naprosyn
COX-2 inhibitors	• Celecoxib			
Opioids	• Butorphanol • Hydrocodone	• Morphine • Oxymorphone	• Demerol	• Oxycodone
Triptans	• Frovatriptan • Rizatriptan	• Sumatriptan	• Naratriptan	• Zolmitriptan
Barbiturates	• Butalbital	• Fiorinal		
Ergotamines	• Dihydroergotamine	• Ergot		

Headache Alert!

Quitting Acute Pain Medication Is Not Easy! During the first month or so after a person abruptly stops taking all acute pain medication for headache pain, the person's headaches will often get worse before they get better. This so-called cold turkey treatment plan is challenging, but it is effective for most people who adhere to it. For many patients, this advice may be a hard pill to swallow (or not swallow, as the case may be); however, in the long run, if they follow the advice they will be rewarded. Studies have shown that approximately 75 percent of patients suffering from rebound headache syndrome will experience dramatic improvement if they can stick to a detoxification plan. There is no sense in trying other treatments until the medications that are causing the problem are stopped, period.

FREQUENTLY ASKED QUESTIONS FOR QUITTING PAIN MEDICATIONS

Which drugs should I stop taking?

The answer is simple: You should stop taking any and all acute pain drugs you are taking. The most common culprit drugs, though, are the OTC medications—the ones most people don't think can be harmful. Still, all medications being taken to treat acute headache pain can and will cause rebound headache syndrome (see Table 5.5).

What Is Considered "Too Much" Medication?

You should take no more than a total of ten doses of acute headache pain medication per month. This does not mean it is okay to take ten Tylenol plus ten Aleve every month. It means that if you add up every time you take any acute pain medication, the total must be less than ten per month—even if you are taking these drugs for pain other than headaches.

How Do I Stop Taking My Medication?

Put simply, there are two options:

- Stop the medications cold turkey.
- Gradually decrease doses until you are no longer taking the medication. Each patient should discuss these options with his or her physician. However, we recommend that patients stop their medication abruptly—as long as it's not an opioid narcotic, since withdrawal from this medication class can be dangerous.

Why Should I Stop Taking My Acute Medication Abruptly?

- The sooner the medications are stopped, the sooner pain relief begins.
- There is a strong behavioral component to rebound headache syndrome. Patients with this condition sometimes can't help themselves from taking their headache pain medication—it almost becomes an anxiety-driven addiction (see "The Behavioral Psychology of Rebound Headache: Pavlov's Dog," opposite page). Thus, if these patients are allowed to gradually reduce their dose, they still have access to their medication and often quickly go back to their old habits, which are causing the problem.

How Long Do I Need to Stop Taking Acute Medication?

After the acute pain medication is stopped (completely) for one to two months, most patients begin to experience significant improvement. As for when you can start using these acute headache medications again, that is not clear, but we recommend at least two to three months of complete abstinence before you start taking these meds again…very carefully!

Individuals with rebound headache syndrome should remember that after stopping medication, their headache pain will likely get worse for several weeks before it begins to get better. But it will get better!

Preventive Headache Medication

Some studies suggest that preventive headache medication will help patients with rebound headache syndrome improve rapidly. However, this will happen only after all of the acute headache pain medication is stopped completely for at least one month.

Headache doctors commonly prescribe preventive migraine medication to patients with rebound headache syndrome (e.g., topiramate, gabapentin, TCAs, and valproic acid). It is important to remember that all of these medications must be taken at a regular daily dosage and may take a few weeks to achieve their full effect. Each of these drugs have specific dosages to treat chronic headache and thus make sure your doctor understands how to use these medications to treat headache.

BOTULINUM TOXINS ALSO SEEM TO WORK

Botox injections, in Dr. Argoff's experience, have been very helpful in reducing rebound headache intensity and severity. Such injections should be given only by a doctor with experience using Botox for this purpose; it is not FDA-approved for this condition, but it has been used in an off-label fashion by headache experts.

The Behavioral Psychology of Rebound Headache: Pavlov's Dog

In some ways, the patient suffering from rebound headache syndrome can be likened to the dog that Russian physiologist Ivan Pavlov used in his classical conditioning experiments. Whenever the patient feels the slightest twinge of head pain, he or she immediately pops a pill to hopefully prevent "the big one" from happening, not knowing that this can lead to yet another problem. While this behavior is quite understandable, it has become part of the problem and needs to be addressed with proper treatment.

Nonmedication Therapies For Rebound Headaches
STRESS MANAGEMENT TECHNIQUES RELIEVE PAIN

One of the most important elements of treating rebound headache syndrome is helping the patient to get rid of the impulse to take medicine at the first feeling of pain. The patient must be taught to use nonmedication treatments, such as relaxation training, therapeutic imagery, and biofeedback, which have all been shown to be effective for the treatment of all types of headaches. Other nonmedication therapies useful in managing rebound headache syndrome are outlined in Table 5.6.

Diagnosing Rebound Headache Syndrome

The neurological examination and laboratory results of patients with rebound headache syndrome are normal. As with chronic tension-type headache, patients with rebound headache syndrome usually have significant tightness and tenderness in the neck and head muscles (myofascial dysfunction). Most headache doctors believe the diagnosis of rebound headache syndrome is fairly simple and can be determined using two criteria (see Table 5.7).

Table 5.6: Nonmedication Therapies Useful for Treating Rebound Headache Syndrome

Acupuncture

Heat treatment

Multidisciplinary headache/pain clinic*

Rehabilitation/PT

TPIs

* Rebound headache syndrome is probably best treated at a multi-disciplinary headache/pain clinic, as it is difficult for patients to stop their acute pain medication and work through the first several weeks of detoxification and worsening pain. Experts at the headache/pain clinic can work together to make the difference between success and failure. Some pain clinics have an inpatient program where you either sleep in the hospital, or sleep in a nearby hotel but go to a daily program that usually consists of educational lectures and PT. Other pain clinics use similar therapies but coordinate separate outpatient appointments.

Rebound Headache Syndrome Explained

Rebound headache syndrome evolves from either migraines or, less commonly, episodic tension-type headaches; for this reason, another name for the condition is *transformed migraine*.

When a patient with migraine or episodic tension-type headaches takes too much acute headache pain medication, rebound headache syndrome will arise. However, interestingly, if people who do not have migraine or episodic tension-type headaches take lots of these same medications, they will not develop rebound headache syndrome, suggesting a genetic factor to this syndrome. Individuals with migraine or tension-type headaches can develop rebound headaches even if they are taking acute medications for other pain conditions, such as arthritis or back pain. It doesn't matter whether the medication is an OTC analgesic, a triptan, an opioid, or a combination of medications; all acute pain medications can cause rebound headache syndrome if taken too frequently by migraine/tension-type headache sufferers.

Table 5.7: Characteristics of Patients with Rebound Headache Syndrome	
The patient with rebound headache syndrome	
1	Has a history of migraine or episodic tension-type headaches and has gradually developed a new type of daily or near-daily headache with features similar to tension-type headaches
AND	
2	During this time has been taking increasing doses of acute pain medication and now is taking daily or near-daily doses of these medications, which are working less and less well over time

ABNORMAL BRAIN PROCESSES IN REBOUND HEADACHE SYNDROME

The underlying changes in the body that cause rebound headache syndrome are unknown. Many experts believe that taking too much acute headache pain medication on a regular basis changes the neurochemicals in the brain of the patient, thereby altering the brain's natural pain system. Most experts also believe that certain muscles can become a secondary source for chronic headaches; anyone who suffers daily head pain will naturally tighten the muscles in his or her head, neck, and shoulders. Eventually, these muscles remain in a tight, stiff, and spastic state, leading to myofascial dysfunction.

CONCLUSION: KNOW YOUR HEADACHE AND SEEK TREATMENT

All types of headaches can be difficult and frustrating to cope with. However, it is important for patients with these conditions to understand what type of headache they have and that help is out there. In many cases, patients can be treated in the primary care setting. When this approach is unsuccessful, most patients will benefit from seeking out a headache specialist or visiting a headache/pain clinic. In the end, patients with headache syndromes should remember that they are not alone and that with the proper treatment they can most often significantly improve their health status and quality of life.

Q & A *with*
Dr. Argoff and Dr. Galer

In patients with migraines, when is it appropriate to prescribe second-line medications, such as barbiturates or short-acting opioids?

These medications should rarely be prescribed. They should be used only infrequently, as "last-resort" options for migraine patients.

How do you manage patients with rebound headache syndrome who cannot resist the urge to continue taking OTC pain medications, even after seeing a pain specialist?

We would first try a very strict schedule of weaning off the medication at home. If the patient is unable to quit this way, then we would recommend a hospital admission to detoxify the patient.

In managing any type of headache, should certain medications be avoided in women who are pregnant? If so, which ones?

Unfortunately, all of the prescription drugs, both acute and preventive medications, should be avoided. Pregnant women should seek out and try nonmedication therapies, all of which can be very effective.

Are there any special techniques for managing patients who have depression associated with their headache condition?

As with all chronic pain conditions, depression is a common problem. It is very important that the depression be treated aggressively with medication. The good news is that many antidepressants have a dual activity whereby they can also treat headaches (even if the patient isn't depressed).

CHAPTER 6

Fighting Fibromyalgia

Holistic therapies provide significant benefit.

the PRESCRIPTION for FIBROMYALGIA

For most patients with fibromyalgia, holistic care is emphasized on a personal basis.

Various medications may be combined with physical therapy (PT) and acupuncture for one person, while massage and medication may be best for another, and aerobic exercise and relaxation therapy may be optimal for a third. Some fibromyalgia patients find relief with biofeedback and cognitive behavioral therapy.

It is important to work with a treatment provider who is willing and able to help you find what is best for you. Stay away from health care providers who make you feel as though you have to justify your pain or seem to disbelieve that you are in pain.

- ✓ Medications
- ✓ Active PT
- ✓ Biofeedback
- ✓ Cognitive behavioral therapy (also called cognitive behavioral treatment)

Debilitating Pain:
A Patient's Story

I'm a thirty-five-year-old, working single mom who for the past year or so has had whole-body pain. It seems like every day I wake up with pain in my legs, arms, and chest or back. I also get headaches all the time. I feel like one big mass of soreness! Also, even when I am able to sleep for six hours, I never feel well rested; I'm just tired all the time. And being a single mom who works, I just can't keep up with all my responsibilities anymore, which makes me depressed and anxious.

Who Gets FMS?

FMS affects approximately ten million people in the United States, and most people who have been diagnosed are female—between 80 percent and 90 percent. Fibromyalgia is one of the most common chronic pain conditions worldwide as well, with an estimated 3 percent to 6 percent of the global population affected. Although it is most prevalent in women, it also affects men and children of all ethnic groups. The diagnosis is usually made between the ages of twenty and fifty years, but the incidence rises with age so that by age eighty, approximately 8 percent of adults meet the American College of Rheumatology diagnostic classification of fibromyalgia.

FMS may occur without any precipitating event; however, it often occurs following a physically or emotionally traumatic event. It is not uncommon, for example, for the first symptoms of fibromyalgia to occur following a motor vehicle accident. In particular, a whiplash-associated injury is more likely to precede the development of fibromyalgia than an injury to the lower extremities; the reason for this is not known.

Symptoms of Fibromyalgia

You have fibromyalgia, with widespread pain in your body, both above and below your waist and on both sides. Typically, on many areas of your body; the joints or skin is sensitive and tender to the touch; these areas are called *tender points*. Fibromyalgia syndrome (FMS) is frequently associated with other symptoms and conditions, such as fatigue, difficulty sleeping, irritable bowel syndrome (IBS), interstitial cystitis (IC, sometimes now termed *painful bladder syndrome*), generalized muscle and joint stiffness especially in the morning, various types of headaches, decreased memory, depression, and anxiety. Keep in mind there is significant variability in the presentation of FMS.

Fibromyalgia Hurts All Over

FMS is characterized by chronic, diffuse pain and multiple tender points throughout the body. Until a few years ago, many doctors believed this condition was mainly due to psychological distress, and too many patients were ignored or were not treated properly. Luckily, with several new drugs approved recently by the FDA to treat FMS, doctors and researchers are finally treating FMS as a serious, biologically based condition, and patients are getting the help they need. Recent research strongly suggests that fibromyalgia is a neurosensory disorder associated with abnormal sensory and pain processing in the central nervous system (brain and spinal cord).

SLEEP DISTURBANCES PREVENT BODILY REST

Sleep disturbance is so common in FMS that at one time, it was believed to be the cause of FMS symptoms. The type of sleep abnormality commonly experienced is often described as nonrestorative sleep, which means you may be able to fall and stay asleep, but when you awaken you do not feel refreshed. If sleeping is a significant problem for you, a sleep specialist evaluation and a formal sleep study may be helpful.

EMOTIONAL STRESS COULD TRIGGER FMS

Some patients who develop fibromyalgia note that their symptoms began following a period of significant emotional stress; for example, following physical, verbal, and/or sexual abuse. People who experience post-traumatic stress disorder (PTSD) are also at risk of developing fibromyalgia. These triggering factors are implicated in the onset of fibromyalgia in genetically predisposed individuals. This means that not all people who experience one of the triggering factors will go on to develop fibromyalgia.

GENETIC FACTORS IN FMS

The disorder is often seen in families, among siblings or among mothers and their children. We are just beginning to understand the genetic factors associated with fibromyalgia. What we do know is that if one person in a family has fibromyalgia, there is an increased likelihood that another close family member will have fibromyalgia compared to an unrelated person.

In addition, genetic associations between fibromyalgia and the way in which the nervous system processes certain neurotransmitters, called *monoamines*, have been noted. Much work remains to better understand the genetic factors associated with fibromyalgia. At present, no good evidence suggests that fibromyalgia is an autoimmune disorder, like rheumatoid arthritis (RA).

Medicines That Treat Fibromyalgia

TRICYCLIC ANTIDEPRESSANTS (TCAS) ARE POWERFUL

There are now three drugs approved by the FDA to treat FMS: pregabalin, duloxetine, and minalcipran. One type of medication that has consistently been found to be useful for FMS include the TCAs, which we believe work mostly by blocking the reuptake of serotonin and norepinephrine in the brain, like the SNRI agents. However, in addition, TCAs can block the activity of another neurotransmitter, acetylcholine, and some actually have local anesthetic-like properties as well. Thus, tricyclics are similar but different from SNRI agents. Amitriptyline and nortriptyline are two examples of TCAs. However, the side effects of TCAs can be significant (see chapter 8).

CYCLOBENZAPRINE IS SIMILAR TO A TCA

The drug cyclobenzaprine is structurally similar to the TCA amitriptyline, but it is marketed as a muscle relaxant. The side effects of cyclobenzaprine are virtually identical to those of amitriptyline and other TCAs. Not all prescribers appear to be aware of the similarity between these two types of medications, and may prescribe both at the same time; don't be afraid to question this as the side effects may be unpleasant if both amitriptyline and cyclobenzaprine are prescribed together.

SSRIs GENERALLY DON'T WORK AS WELL

Serotonin-specific reuptake inhibiting (SSRI) medications such as fluoxetine and sertraline inhibit the reuptake of serotonin, increasing the amount available in the brain. None of the medications in this category are FDA-approved for the treatment of fibromyalgia. In our experience and that of others, they are not as effective as TCAs for reducing pain if you have fibromyalgia. Nevertheless, some people may find an SSRI medication to be very effective for their fibromyalgia.

Get the Facts about Fibromyalgia

- FMS is the most common widespread chronic pain disorder lasting three months or longer.
- FMS can be reliably diagnosed and treated with effective strategies.
- FMS may be associated with other conditions such as RA, depression, painful bladder syndrome (IC), and migraine headaches.
- FMS may be associated with sleep difficulty, problems with thinking, and morning stiffness.

121

What's New: FDA-Approved Drugs for FMS

Over the past few years the FDA has approved several medications for the treatment of FMS, including pregabalin (Lyrica), duloxetine (Cymbalta), and minalcipran (Savella).

How do they work? Pregabalin is considered an anticonvulsant/neuromodulator, which means it can reduce the excitability of the nerves that may be associated with the signs and symptoms of fibromyalgia. Its proposed mechanism of action, based on a great deal of scientific research, is that it blocks calcium from entering an active nerve cell in the central nervous system, limiting its ability to be as excitable or "ornery" as it would be otherwise.

Duloxetine and minalcipran are both serotonergic noradrenergic reuptake inhibiting (SNRI) drugs that have also been shown to help people who are depressed. The proposed mechanism of their pain-reducing effects is through their effect on two nerve chemicals (neurotransmitters): serotonin and norepinephrine. These SNRI medications prevent the reuptake of both serotonin and norepinephrine in the brain, resulting in a greater amount of each available. Since these neurotransmitters dampen pain signals through nerve pathways

(continued)

122

OTHER DRUGS THAT ARE WORTH TRYING

Certain medications such as tizanidine, baclofen, and nonsteroidal anti-inflammatory drugs (NSAIDs) have not been as carefully studied for use with FMS—or have been studied with mixed, conflicting results.

Tizanidine Helps with Spasticity

Tizanidine has been studied outside the United States for decades for a variety of painful conditions including low back pain and facial pain. In the United States, it is FDA-approved only for the treatment of spasticity (increased muscle tone after injury to the spinal cord or brain). Other studies in painful conditions in the United States have shown that it can be effective for people with chronic headaches. Tizanidine inhibits the release of certain neurotransmitters that can excite the nervous system, but the exact mechanism for its role in reducing pain is not known. Side effects include sedation, dizziness, and dry mouth.

Baclofen May Sometimes Help

Baclofen is also a medication that is FDA-approved in the United States for spasticity and has been studied in certain pain states including trigeminal neuralgia. Its mechanism of action is through the GABA receptor. GABA is another neurotransmitter in the central nervous system, but instead of exciting the nervous system, it actually inhibits it. Again, like most medications used to treat pain, the exact mechanism of how it works to relieve pain is unknown. Side effects of baclofen include drowsiness, dizziness, weakness, headache, nausea, constipation, and diarrhea.

NSAIDs Have Limited Success with FMS

Although there is no evidence that fibromyalgia is associated with active inflammation, NSAIDs have been used to treat fibromyalgia with limited success in some people. Note the potential harmful side effects of NSAIDs if overused!

Nonmedication Treatments For FMS

Nonmedication treatments for FMS are at least as important as medications, if not more so. Therefore, it is vital that you find a doctor who is familiar with all of these nondrug therapies so that he or she can find the best one for you.

ACTIVE PT IS CRITICAL

One of the most important components of every FMS patient's treatment is an active PT program. Keeping your body in good physical shape is critical to treating the pain and disability associated with FMS. You can do this by enrolling in an active PT program, swimming, walking, biking, or whatever other form of exercise you feel comfortable doing. Aerobic exercise may strengthen your muscles, helping you to feel less weakness and stiffness. This may be especially helpful in the morning when so many fibromyalgia patients experience muscle stiffness. As you become stronger, physical activity may be less likely to cause injuries. Many people find that after participating in aerobic exercises for a while, they see an improvement in their ability to fall asleep and stay asleep.

Aerobic exercise is also known to stimulate the release of our body's natural pain relievers, or endorphins. Finally, the overall health benefits of aerobic exercise, including with respect to cardiovascular illness, should also be remembered.

Some people are more likely to follow an exercise regime if they exercise with a group as opposed to alone, so look for a group exercise program if this pertains to you. Unless you are already an active exerciser, begin to gradually include an aerobic exercise program into your treatment regimen. You don't want to overdo it, especially at the beginning. Start with only five minutes per day and build to thirty or so minutes per day, several days per week. Warm up by stretching for a few minutes before starting your exercise. It is normal to feel increased soreness at the beginning of any exercise program, but the good news is that as you continue to exercise, this will likely be replaced with the benefits we noted earlier. Always remember to allow time for rest after an exercise session. How long should you keep this up? For as long as you can!

PASSIVE PT PROVIDES TEMPORARY RELIEF

Though definitely a secondary treatment, sometimes passive PT modalities such as therapeutic massage, transcutaneous electrical nerve stimulation (TENS), and hydrotherapy may provide temporary relief of the pain associated with fibromyalgia. However, these should never be a replacement for an active PT program, as your goal is to become more active and functional, and using passive approaches alone is less likely to produce this result.

(What's New: continued)

that travel from the brain to the spinal cord, the increased amount of them can lead to reduced pain.

What are the side effects? All these medications have very good clinical trial data demonstrating that they can be very helpful compared to placebos in treating FMS symptoms, with tolerable side effects for most patients.

The most common side effects of pregabalin (Lyrica) are dizziness, somnolence, dry mouth, swelling of the lower extremities, blurred vision, weight gain, and abnormal thinking. Pregabalin is also considered an antiseizure medication, and antiseizure medications are known to slightly increase the risk of suicidal thoughts and behavior in people taking them for *any* reason.

The most common side effects of duloxetine (Cymbalta) are nausea, increased sweating, dizziness, constipation, dry mouth, sleepiness, and decreased appetite.

The most common side effects of milnacipran (Savella) are nausea, headache, constipation, dizziness, insomnia, hot flashes, increased sweating, vomiting, palpitations, increased heart rate, dry mouth, and high blood pressure. Both duloxetine and milnacipran, as SNRI agents, are also associated with the risk of increased suicidal thoughts and behavior in children, teens, and young adults.

FMS Alert!

Opioids May Cause More Pain
The role of opioid pain relievers for FMS is unclear and somewhat controversial. This may sound counterintuitive; after all, aren't opioid medications used to treat all forms of moderate to severe chronic pain, and doesn't fibromyalgia cause moderate to severe chronic pain? Let's first acknowledge that opioids are known to be associated with abuse and misuse, and of course, we need to be concerned about prescribing opioids carefully to maximize benefit and minimize harm. In previous animal experiments and in recent human experiments, it is becoming increasingly recognized that use of opioids in some individuals may be associated with increased pain, a concept known as *opioid-induced hyperalgesia* (excessive pain).

Although this does not appear to occur in most patients and health care providers can monitor for this, using a type of medication that could itself cause even further pain to FMS patients, even if only occasionally, is certainly not ideal. Much research is underway to further examine this observed potential effect.

Therapeutic Massage Encourages Natural Painkillers

Massage therapy can reduce pain, stiffness, and the number of tender points associated with fibromyalgia. Although not known for sure, it is thought that massage therapy works by encouraging the body's release of serotonin, norepinephrine, and endorphins. Swedish massage, deep tissue massage, and myofascial release massage are different types of massage; however, no clear study has been conducted that compares these massage types and their effectiveness in reducing fibromyalgia pain.

TENS Is Portable

TENS is a noninvasive means to treat fibromyalgia pain. Each TENS unit comes with a battery, electrodes, and an electric signal generator. The electrodes are often on felt or rubber pads and are placed on the painful area(s) of your body. When the electric signal generator is turned on, nerves in the skin and muscles are electrically stimulated, and pain transmission may be dampened, resulting in pain relief. The exact mechanism of action of TENS is not known. The TENS unit can be used several times daily, or less frequently for an indefinite period of time. Many people first learn about TENS when working with a physical therapist; if helpful, TENS units can be purchased or rented for home use.

Hydrotherapy Helps, Hot or Cold

Also known as *balneotherapy*, the use of hydrotherapy for pain reduction has been noted for hundreds of years. Water in various forms, from ice to steam, may be used to help reduce pain. Use of ice, compresses (hot or cold), and baths (hot or cold) are some types of hydrotherapy that may be helpful.

BIOFEEDBACK PUTS YOU IN CONTROL OF STRESS

Biofeedback works by teaching you to not only recognize your body's reaction to stress, but also alter its reaction to stress to result in less pain. For example, stress may increase your heart rate, which may be associated with other effects such as increased pain. A biofeedback machine can inform you through lights or sound when your heart rate is increasing so that you can learn how to limit this, and thus limit the pain. Different types of biofeedback are available which monitor different body functions including muscle activity (electromyography biofeedback) and skin temperature (peripheral skin temperature biofeedback).

COGNITIVE BEHAVIORAL THERAPY CHANGES YOUR THINKING

Cognitive behavioral therapy is a type of psychotherapy. It is centered on your recognition that how you think about something strongly influences how you feel and act. Cognitive therapy is focused on helping you to change the way certain thoughts influence your symptoms, and behavioral therapy focuses on reducing the behaviors that cause the symptoms. It is well known that fibromyalgia symptoms can be worsened by stress and other emotions. Cognitive behavioral therapy can help you to manage this in a way that may result in modification of certain behaviors and reduced pain severity. A psychotherapist will work with you to help accomplish this.

VITAMIN AND HERBAL SUPPLEMENTS

There have been many claims regarding the role of vitamin and herbal supplements for treatment of fibromyalgia. The jury is still out as to whether there is any truth to these claims; however, many people commonly use vitamin and herbal supplements for their treatment. These include S-adenosylmethionine (SAMe), magnesium, vitamin D, 5-hydroxytryptophan (5-HTP), and vitamin B_{12}. As always, we recommend that you discuss optimal therapies and doses with your doctor.

Diagnosing Fibromyalgia

In 1990, rheumatology experts who were seeing many patients with widespread pain but who did not have another rheumatologic condition to explain it met and agreed on the criteria for diagnosing FMS. As you can see, the diagnosis is based only on patient symptoms and a doctor's examination. More recently, published guidelines from the American Pain Society focus on other steps to complete in the evaluation of a person with suspected FMS: A complete history and physical examination needs to be completed, with special attention paid to medical conditions that may mimic or exacerbate FMS. Laboratory tests (see below) need to be considered and completed to rule-out these other conditions that may mimic FMS.

THE DEFINITION OF A TENDER POINT

Tender points are defined as locations experiencing tenderness when approximately 9 lbs (4 kg) of pressure is exerted at them. Nine pounds of pressure is the amount required to blanch (turn white) your thumbnail when pressure is applied.

What's New: Sodium Oxybate May Help FMS Patients

A medication that is under active investigation as a treatment for fibromyalgia but at the time of this writing is FDA-approved for only certain sleep-related disorders is sodium oxybate (Xyrem). Since this medication may help to prolong stage III/IV sleep—so called restorative sleep—and since such sleep is often disrupted in patients with fibromyalgia, this may be an effective treatment. Initial study results are encouraging; however, because there is a potential for abuse and dependence as well as for use for nonmedical situations (this drug is actually the "date rape drug"), even if it is approved for fibromyalgia there will likely be significant restrictions regarding its use.

Let's review the nine tender point locations, starting with the top of your body, keeping in mind that these locations are for each side of your body (bilateral). The **occiput** location is at the back of your skull. The **lower cervical location** is in the anterior region, overlapping the fifth through seventh cervical vertebrae. Imagine putting your hands on the side of your neck and moving them down until you hit your collarbone (clavicle). This is where the lower cervical location is. The **trazpezius** location is where someone who is massaging your shoulders would be placing his or her thumbs. The **second rib** location is just under the collarbone and just lateral to (to the side of) the sternum. The **supraspinatus** location is at the top of what you would typically call your shoulder blade. The **lateral epicondyle** location is at the general level of the elbow on the thumb side of the region. The **gluteal area** location is in the upper outer area of your buttocks. The **greater trochanteric** location in plain terms is the area around your hips just underneath the buttocks. The **knee** location is the "inside" aspect of your knee.

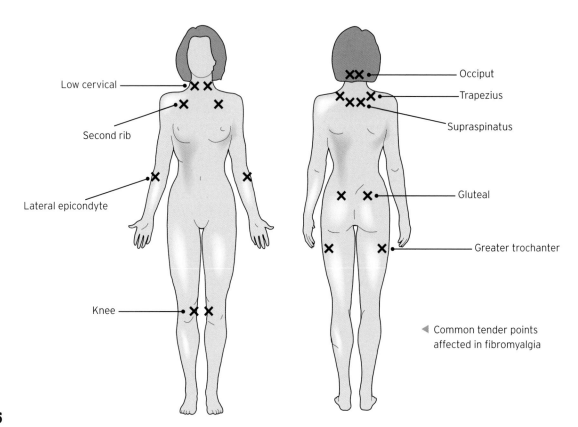

◀ Common tender points affected in fibromyalgia

It is very important to note that FMS "Tender Points" are very different than Myofascial Dysfunction "Trigger Points." FMS Tender Points are at well-defined areas in the body, whereas myofascial Trigger Points can be located within any muscle, ligament or tendon. Also Trigger Points are actually felt as tight hard knots, whereas typically Tender Points do not have any palpable node when pressed.

LABORATORY TESTS ARE NOT REVEALING

As with most other chronic pain conditions, there are no characteristic laboratory abnormalities for FMS. This includes X-ray, CT scan, and MRI findings. This means that all of the tests your doctor orders will likely be normal, but you still may have FMS. Why do doctors order these tests if nothing shows up? Often, doctors use laboratory tests to rule out other medical conditions that can be associated with widespread pain, such as RA and other conditions, as we summarize later in this chapter.

Fibromyalgia Explained

Fibromyalgia most often presents in a young or middle-aged female as chronic, widespread pain. Recent studies and emerging medical evidence increasingly point to dysfunction of the central nervous system (brain and spinal cord) as a major reason why FMS occurs. These studies suggest that a number of triggering factors, such as medical illness, emotional stress, or physical stress (following surgery or trauma), produce abnormal central nervous system processing, resulting in central sensitization. This literally means that the central nervous system facilitates the transmission and processing of especially painful sensations, and is why a normally nonpainful sensation can be experienced as painful by someone with FMS. Basically, it's like your brain has turned up the volume with regards to how it perceives pain signals coming from your body. Whereas a non-FMS person will experience a dull ache from a sore muscle and perceive it as "mild and bothersome but not painful," the exact same signal in a FMS patient will have her or his brain perceive it as "severe and intolerable pain."

Genetic factors have been suggested as being important, since not all people who are subjected to the known triggering factors for FMS experience this syndrome, and because several studies have noted that if you have FMS, close family members are much more likely to develop FMS than others without family members who have FMS.

What's New: Acupuncture to Treat Fibromyalgia

Several recent studies have emphasized the potential benefit of acupuncture for people with fibromyalgia. The best results have been in reducing fatigue and anxiety levels associated with FMS.

Examination Findings: FMS

The only important finding on examination is the identification of tender points throughout the body in specific regions. Other than the presence of multiple tender points, the rest of the FMS patient's examination should be completely normal, unless the person with FMS is also affected by another condition at the same time, in which an abnormal examination would be expected (e.g., RA and FMS).

Other scientific evidence has given us a set of clues as to what is causing and contributing to these changes in the brain and spinal cord causing central sensitization, including the observation that certain nerve chemicals (neurotransmitters) that are responsible for pain transmission are seen in higher concentrations in FMS patients compared to nonaffected individuals. These nerve chemicals include substance P, glutamate, and brain-derived neurotropic factor. Abnormalities in serotonin and norepinephrine, two nerve chemicals highly responsible for many functions in the central nervous system, including mood and pain control, have also been noted in FMS patients and these are believed to significantly contribute to the development and maintenance of FMS. Abnormalities of the neurotransmitter dopamine are also being studied in FMS.

The diagnosis of FMS may be delayed in some instances as the initial symptoms may be different from person to person. It is important that the person who is evaluating you is trained to recognize FMS. You can contact the National Fibromyalgia Association to find an experienced practitioner in your area.

SYNDROMES ASSOCIATED WITH FIBROMYALGIA

Fibromyalgia is associated with a number of other syndromes, often referred to as the *comorbidities of fibromyalgia*. These include chronic fatigue syndrome, IBS, IC (painful bladder syndrome), migraines and other types of headaches, restless legs syndrome, difficulty with memory and thinking in general, skin abnormalities such as sensitivities to various substances and rashes, a variety of psychiatric syndromes, dry eyes and dry mouth, sleep disturbances, Raynaud's disease, dizziness, ringing in the ears, and difficulty with vision. We describe several of these in this section.

In addition to the overlap with other syndromes, fibromyalgia may coexist with certain other specific illnesses such as systemic lupus erythematosus, RA, chronic Lyme disease, chronic hepatitis C infection, and many others.

Chronic Fatigue Syndrome Affects Different Systems

Chronic fatigue syndrome is an ongoing disorder defined by severe and chronic fatigue. This disorder may affect a number of different body systems, and thus many other symptoms may occur in addition to fatigue. Some of these symptoms include sleep difficulties, fatigue, muscle pain, and difficulty with thinking. Chronic fatigue syndrome can last for several months, or unfortunately for some, for years.

IBS Produces Diarrhea and Constipation

IBS is a chronic condition that affects the bowel, medically known as the large intestine. Symptoms include diarrhea and constipation. There is no clear structural or chemical cause for the syndrome. According to some reports, up to 70 percent of people with fibromyalgia experience IBS as well. As with fibromyalgia, women are more often affected than men.

Restless Legs Syndrome Keeps People Awake

Restless legs syndrome is a neurological disorder in which the affected person experiences unpleasant and sometimes painful sensations in the legs, along with an uncontrollable urge to move when resting to relieve these feelings. Restless legs syndrome sensations are often described by people as burning, unpleasant, creeping, or tugging. Some people with restless legs syndrome describe the sensation as though insects are crawling inside their legs. Lying down or trying to relax actually promotes the symptoms, clearly disrupting the ability to sleep. Even people with restless legs syndrome alone report impaired memory or difficulty concentrating, so one should realize how experiencing both restless legs syndrome and fibromyalgia may magnify the severity of these problems.

IC Causes Pain in the Bladder Region

IC (interstitial cystitis) is a medical condition associated with discomfort or pain in the bladder and the neighboring pelvic region. The symptoms vary considerably from person to person, from mild to severe discomfort to excruciating pain, pressure, or tenderness in the bladder and pelvic area. Patients may complain of an urgent need to urinate, a frequent need to urinate, or both. Pain may change in intensity as the bladder fills with urine or after it is emptied following urination. Women's symptoms often get worse during menstruation, and women may sometimes experience pain during vaginal intercourse. IC is more common in women than in men.

TMJ Involves Pain in the Jaw

Temporomandibular joint dysfunction, also known as temporomandibular joint syndrome (TMJ), refers to a group of painful medical conditions involving the jaw and the temporomandibular joint. Muscles involved in chewing are also responsible for opening and closing the mouth. The jawbone is controlled by the temporomandibular joint, and proper movement of the temporomandibular joint is required for sufficient opening and proper closing of the mouth. Proper functioning of the temporomandibular joint also allows you to talk, chew, and yawn.

Raynaud's Disease Makes Toes and Nose Cold

Raynaud's disease is a condition that results in some body areas, especially the fingers, toes, tip of your nose, and ears, to feel numb and cool in response to cold temperatures, stress, and other triggers. In Raynaud's disease, smaller arteries that supply blood to your skin suddenly narrow, limiting blood circulation to affected areas. Raynaud's disease is the term used to describe this condition when there is no known cause; Raynaud's phenomenon is the term used to describe this condition when there is a known cause. Known causes include scleroderma, lupus, certain medications (e.g., beta blockers), carpal tunnel syndrome, thyroid abnormalities, and RA. It is estimated that between 30 percent and 50 percent of people with fibromyalgia experience Raynaud's phenomenon.

Mood Disorders Are Prevalent with FMS

Mood disorders are commonly experienced by people with fibromyalgia, with bipolar disorder and major depressive disorder the most commonly experienced. Other psychiatric conditions that may be experienced by people with fibromyalgia include generalized anxiety disorder, obsessive-compulsive disorder, PTSD, social phobias, and eating disorders.

The Natural Course Of Fibromyalgia

Even though significant progress has been made in understanding FMS, fibromyalgia remains a challenging condition to treat. The excellent news is that many clinical studies show that FMS patients can be effectively evaluated and diagnosed and that they can reduce their symptoms through a variety of treatment options. The FDA has recently approved three medications for FMS, and much more medical research is underway for other treatments. Partnering with well-informed health care professionals, FMS patients can expect to experience notable improvement in their symptoms and quality of life. Developing an individualized treatment plan that identifies effective treatment approaches to making necessary lifestyle changes that are best for you is necessary for success.

CONCLUSION: FMS IS GAINING UNDERSTANDING AND TREATMENT

The diagnosis of FMS should be considered in all people with long-standing (chronic), widespread pain. Numerous advances in our understanding of potential mechanisms of FMS have been made. Many effective treatments for FMS—both medication-based and nonmedication-based—are currently available. Recently, three medications for FMS have been approved by the FDA, and many others are currently being studied. FMS patients should be empowered by these positive developments.

I am a thirty-eight-year-old woman and I suffered a whiplash injury when I was involved in a car accident last year. I am feeling pain throughout my body, but all tests are normal and my primary care doctor says there is nothing wrong with me other than normal aches and pains. I was sent to a rheumatologist and an orthopedist, and they each suggested that I was exaggerating my symptoms and did not suggest any treatment. Over-the-counter medications don't help, and I cannot comfortably exercise because of the pain. I cannot sleep well, and it is becoming more difficult for me to take care of my family and work as a teacher. What should I do?

You need to contact the National Fibromyalgia Association (Dr. Argoff is a member of the Medical Advisory Board of this association) to find a physician who is well informed regarding FMS and who practices where you live. In our experience, the diagnosis of FMS is often delayed, and as a result, people suffer. Studies have suggested that some people with FMS had to see as many as seventeen doctors before being properly diagnosed with FMS. Stay calm and find the right person to evaluate and treat you, and hopefully soon you will be better!

I am a fifty-eight-year-old woman who has been diagnosed with FMS. I have been prescribed pregabalin (Lyrica) for this, and in addition, I exercise regularly and meditate frequently. I am too sleepy when I take the pregabalin as prescribed (225 mg by mouth twice daily); it's helping my pain, but I cannot function during the day because I am so tired. My doctor says this is normal, but what can I do? Should I take a stimulant with it?

We have found sedation to be one of the most common side effects of pregabalin, one of the FDA-approved medications for FMS. There are several options for you to consider. First, consider asking your doctor if it is acceptable to take more pregabalin at night before you go to sleep and less during the day, so the sedation would be heavier when you are going to sleep (that would be good!) and lighter when you want to be active. If that is not effective, consider reducing the dose of pregabalin under your doctor's guidance and ask about additional medical options. For example, adding duloxetine (Cymbalta) to your treatment regimen may enhance your overall response and not cause any additional sedation. Work with your doctor, as there are many treatment combinations to consider. Don't be discouraged!

CHAPTER 7

Overcoming Cancer Pain

A multi-treatment approach is

necessary for significant relief.

Residual Pain after Cancer Treatment:
A Patient's Story

I am a forty-eight-year-old female with breast cancer that has spread to my bones and liver. I had previously undergone a radical mastectomy, and then a few years later I learned that the cancer had spread to my bones and liver. After being treated with chemotherapy and radiation, it appears that the cancer is under control, but my lower back kills me and my feet are numb and always burning. I am glad that the cancer is under control, but I am still suffering in pain.

the PRESCRIPTION *for* CANCER PAIN

The main types of cancer-related pain treatment include pharmacologic, interventional, physical, and complementary therapies.

Depending on the type of pain you are experiencing, one or several of these treatments in combination may be of benefit. It is important to note that because cancer-related pain can be caused by so many different reasons, an evaluation by a knowledgeable doctor is even more important than with other pain conditions.

- ✓ Medications
- ✓ Interventions (nerve blocks, intravenous infusions, and intrathecal medications)
- ✓ Physical therapy (PT)
- ✓ Complementary therapies such as acupuncture

Symptoms of Cancer Pain

You have cancer-related pain. Since the causes of such pain are many and any part of the body may be involved, basically all types of pain qualities may be experienced (dull ache, burning, shooting, electric shocks, etc.). And because the cancer itself, a cancer metastasis, or treatments can affect all areas of the body, virtually all regions of your body can develop cancer-related pain. Also, remember that having cancer does not prevent you from developing "non-cancer related" pain conditions, such as migraines, tension headaches, arthritis, myofascial back pain, or neck pain. If you have "cancer pain" then probably the most important thing you can do is have a good oncologist and a pain doctor so they can determine the correct diagnosis and treatments for your pain.

Cancer pain may have both a persistent baseline quality present continuously or nearly continuously as well as superimposed breakthrough episodes of pain. You need to assess and discuss both components with your doctor. Breakthrough pain is infrequent and occurs seemingly out of the blue, or may be associated with movement (incident pain), or may occur just before the next dose of pain medication is to be given. Both the baseline pain and the breakthrough pain must be properly assessed and treated for the best outcome to occur. Keep in mind that most patients with cancer pain will experience both underlying, near-constant pain and episodes of breakthrough pain.

Hope For Cancer Patients

Millions of Americans experience various types of cancer and many will experience cancer-related pain. Fortunately, a multitude of treatments are available for cancer-related pains; however, regretably, even today cancer pain remains too frequently undertreated. Realistically, cancer-related pain cannot always be completely eliminated; however, most people with cancer-related pain should expect that their symptoms will be significantly controlled. Many therapies, both medication-based and nonmedication-based, are available to properly and optimally treat cancer-related pain. However, certain barriers to the best available cancer-pain management still exist: The health care provider may not be up to speed; the health care system in general causes obstacles. Therefore, it is important that the patient or a loved one be assertive about receiving the best possible care.

Cancer Pain Alert!

Your Involvement Is Critical
The key to optimal management of all cancer-related pain is an approach that stresses the involvement of the person with the pain! Take notes about your pain to tell and discuss with your doctor(s):

- Where is it?
- How often does it occur?
- How would you describe the quality of the pain?
- What makes your pain worse?
- What makes your pain better?
- Do you have any other symptoms?

Remember that the best pain management requires a team approach among the patient, family, and health care provider.

Get the Facts: Most Common Cancer-Related Pains

Some are caused by tumor invasion of pain-sensitive structures:

- Into bone
- Into nerve
- Into organs (colon, stomach, liver)

Others are caused by complications of cancer therapies:

- Post-surgery (nerve injury, scarring)
- Chemotherapy
- Radiation therapy

Medications That Treat Cancer Pain

Many years ago, the World Health Organization proposed a three-step medication "ladder" to be considered for all types of cancer pain (see figure 7.1). This step-wise or ladder approach is based on the use of less potent medications for milder pain (step 1), more potent medications for moderately severe pain (step 2), and the most potent medications for the most severe pain (step 3).

Keep in mind that this ladder approach should be used only as a guide; if a person with cancer pain initially experiences severe pain, that person does not need to be first treated with less potent (steps 1 and then 2) approaches before receiving a more appropriate treatment for the pain. After being evaluated by his/her doctor, a person with severe cancer-related pain may often best be helped by going directly to step 3.

HOW ARE MEDICATIONS BEST TAKEN?

Medication can be taken in many different ways to treat cancer-related pain (called *routes of administration*). Medications can be taken orally in pill, tablet, or capsule form; through the skin by patch, gel, cream, liquid, or injection; through a rectal route as a suppository; or through an intraspinal route.

The timing of when you take the medications can be either as needed (PRN) or around the clock (ATC). Different approaches work best for different people with cancer pain; what is most important is that the doctor and the patient are able to communicate effectively to arrive at the best approach for that person.

NONSTEROIDAL ANTI-INFLAMMATORY DRUGS (NSAIDS) AND ACETAMINOPHEN

NSAIDs include agents such as ibuprofen, naproxen, diclofenac, and many others. Acetaminophen is the generic term for the active ingredient in Tylenol. These medications may be useful for mild to moderate pain. Also, these drugs may sometimes be used in combination with an opioid medication, such as in Percocet, Vicodin, or Vicoprofen, which often is a very effective combination for many patients.

NSAIDs and acetaminophen are available as oral tablets, capsules, liquid preparations, and suppositories. One NSAID, ketorolac, is available through intravenous or intramuscular injection. Recently the FDA also approved an intravenous form of ibuprofen and is currently reviewing to see whether an intravenous form of acetaminophen will be approved for availability in the United States.

Since many NSAIDs, as well as acetaminophen, are available as nonprescription (over-the-counter) and prescription medications (acetaminophen is an ingredient of many combination drugs such as Percocet and Vicodin), the patient must be very careful about not using an excessive amount of these medications by accident. Always ask your health care provider and pharmacist about safe dosing of these drugs.

Opioids For Cancer Pain

Opioids are a type of pain reliever typically used in the management of moderate to severe pain. Medications in this category include morphine, codeine, hydromorphone, hydrocodone, methadone, oxycodone, oxymorphone, levorphanol, and fentanyl. Each works slightly differently in the nervous system (brain and spinal cord pain regions). Because each person has a slightly different response to opioid medications, what works best for one patient may be different from what works best for another.

Opioids are considered and chosen based on how quickly they act and for how long, which depends on which ingredients are used to make the pill or patch. Although one opioid type of medication may start working within fifteen minutes

Figure 7.1: World Health Organizations Analgesic Ladder

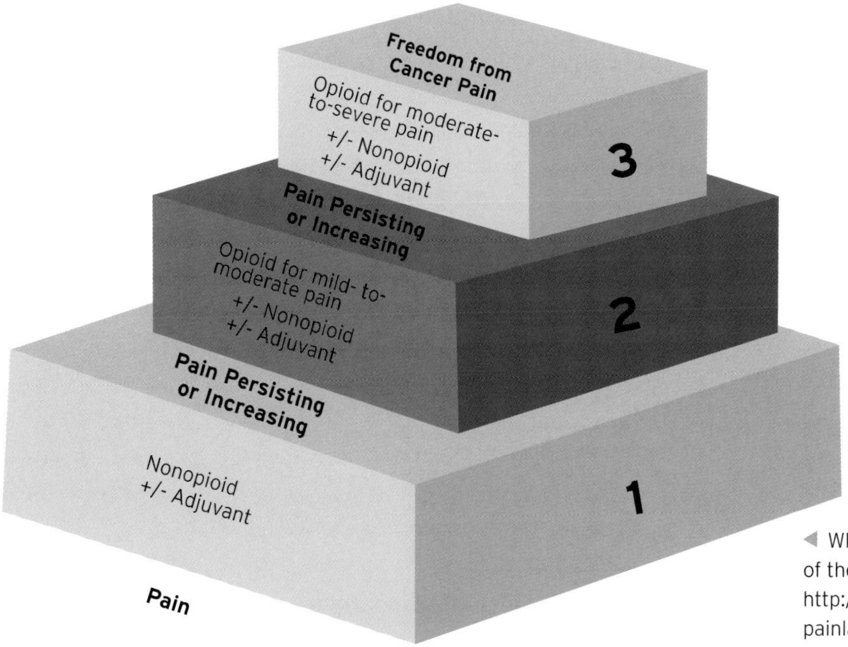

◀ WHO's Pain Relief Ladder, courtesy of the World Health Organization, http://www.who.int/cancer/palliative/painladder/en

Cancer Alert!

New Back Pain Is a Medical Emergency for Cancer Patients
If you have cancer and you suddenly develop back pain or a new type of back pain, it is a medical emergency. This might mean you have a metastasis in your vertebra (back bone; see X-ray on page 149). Why is that a medical emergency? Because if the tumor grows, it may suddenly choke off your spinal cord and result in leg weakness and bowel/bladder incontinence (called *spinal cord compression*). If this occurs and it is not treated immediately, such problems can become permanent. It is very important to let your doctor know right away or for you to immediately go to an emergency department for evaluation if you suddenly develop back pain or a new type of back pain.

Cancer Alert!

Use NSAIDs with Caution

Patients with cancer often have problems with blood clotting; NSAIDs can inhibit platelets, the component in the blood that helps blood to clot. Therefore, these medications should be used carefully in patients with cancer-related pain. Other important side effects of NSAIDs include ulcers, liver and kidney problems, and cardiovascular complications including heart attacks. Though acetaminophen is not considered an NSAID, excessive use of this medication on a regular basis can lead to liver and kidney problems as well. And because many cancer patients are prone to liver and kidney problems, acetaminophen also should be used cautiously in many patients with cancer-related pain.

and wear off within a few hours, others may take longer to begin working—perhaps an hour—but may last half the day. Whereas one drug may contain an opioid as its sole ingredient, others combine an opioid with a nonopioid medication—for example, acetaminophen or ibuprofen. One is not necessarily better than another, so work with your doctor to find the best option if an opioid is to be prescribed for you.

Some opioid medications are designed to be effective quickly and wear off within a few hours. These are short-acting or immediate-release opioids. Several short-acting opioids have a particularly rapid onset of action, and are known as *rapid-onset opioids*. These potent medications are generally used for management of breakthrough pain. Other opioid medications take longer to begin working, but also last longer. These opioid formulations are called *long-acting* or *extended-release opioids*.

For a person with persistent cancer-related pain, the long-acting opioids may be considered ideal, since they need to be taken less frequently than would an equivalent amount of short-acting medication. Also, if taken regularly as directed, long-acting opioids keep a steady pain-relieving amount of the medication in your blood, even when you sleep. Many cancer-related pain patients are best managed with a combination of both long-acting and short-acting opioids because in addition to persistent pain, there may be episodes of breakthrough pain requiring additional treatment. At times, cancer pain may be effectively managed with short-acting opioids only.

TRAMADOL COMBINES THE ACTION OF A TRICYCLIC ANTIDEPRESSANT (TCA) AND OPIOID

Tramadol and its metabolite together have dual mechanisms for pain relief, including acting like a TCA and a weak opioid. Although it is not as potent as medications such as morphine, many people who use tramadol find that it is helpful. It is available in both short- and long-acting forms.

SPINAL OPIOIDS AS A LAST RESORT

Opioid medication can be directly injected into the fluid around the spinal cord in a procedure called an intraspinal injection. The use of intraspinal medications on a long-term basis requires outpatient surgery to place an implantable device (a pump) that serves as a reservoir for the medication that will be pumped through a catheter directly into the intraspinal space. This treatment is clearly reserved only for patients with cancer-related pain who have been unable to benefit from oral, intravenous, intramuscular, topical, and transdermal drugs.

Common Opioid Side Effects

Regardless of which opioid is prescribed and regardless of whether it is a short-acting or long-acting formulation, all opioid medications commonly cause side effects. Side effects of opioids need to be anticipated and treated. The most common side effects are constipation, nausea, vomiting, and sleepiness. Opioid-induced constipation is common, occurring in as many as 70 percent of the people treated with these types of medications. Fortunately, many treatments are available to address the constipation.

Nausea and vomiting occurs in between one-third and two-thirds of the people using opioids for cancer-related pain. If this does occur, it usually goes away fairly quickly—within the first week of treatment. It appears that our body "gets used" to this effect of the medication and it often stops being a problem. On the other hand, for reasons that are not clear constipation does not go away most of the time, making it challenging to continue to use an opioid. Many medical treatments are available to help reduce the nausea and lessen the likelihood of vomiting. Collectively, these medications are known as anti-emetics.

Other, less-common opioid side effects include difficulty thinking, hallucinations, delirium, reduced sexual function, and an increase—not a decrease—in pain. Also, it has been shown that chronic opioid treatment may result in reduced testosterone levels in men and a loss of menstruation in women. Since sexuality is a part of the normal quality of life for many people, this is an adverse effect. If this happens to you, be sure to communicate this to your health care provider, as there is treatment! Treatment can include changing the type of opioid used, using nonopioid medications, or hormonal replacement (if medically acceptable and not otherwise contraindicated). Dry mouth, difficulty urinating, itchy skin (most often due to the release of histamine by an opioid and not an allergic reaction to the opioid, but check with your health care provider), sleep disturbances, and depression may occur as well.

If a person is prescribed an opioid for cancer-pain management, that person must agree to follow the way the drug has been prescribed. Do not take more or

Types of Opioids

Immediate-Release Opioids
- Morphine (e.g., Roxanol, MSIR)
- Codeine
- Codeine and acetaminophen (e.g., Tylenol with Codeine)
- Fentanyl (rapid onset; e.g., Actiq, Fentora, Onsolis)
- Oxycodone (e.g., Roxicodone)
- Oxycodone + acetaminophen (e.g., Percocet)
- Oxymorphone (e.g., Opana IR)
- Hydrocodone
- Hydrocodone and acetaminophen (e.g., Lortab, Norco, Vicodin)
- Hydrocodone and ibuprofen (e.g., Vicoprofen)
- Hydromorphone (e.g., Dilaudid)
- Tapentadol (e.g., Nucynta)
- Tramadol (e.g., Ultram)
- Tramadol and acetaminophen (e.g., Ultracet)

Extended-Release Opioids
- Morphine (e.g., Morphine ER, MS Contin, Avinza, Kadian, Embeda)
- Oxymorphone (e.g., Opana ER)
- Fentanyl (e.g., Fentanyl Patch, Duragesic)
- Oxycodone (e.g., Oxycodone ER, Oxycontin)
- Methadone
- Levorphanol
- Tramadol (e.g., Ultram ER, Ryzolt)

139

Special Words about Methadone

Although many associate methadone with the treatment of drug addiction, in fact it was originally developed in Germany during World War II to treat pain and other disorders, and can be an excellent pain reliever for some patients. Methadone can be administered orally, through injection, and rectally. However, methadone is somewhat unpredictable with respect to its effect from person to person, so it should be prescribed only by doctors who are experienced in its use. It can interact with many other medications, foods, and herbs, and may cause serious cardiac side effects, including death.

On the other hand, certain features of methadone may render it more effective for certain types of pain (neuropathic) compared to other opioids. Methadone has a nonopioid mechanism in addition to being an opioid, making it almost like two medications in one pill; however, it is among the most difficult medications to prescribe unless the prescriber has appropriate knowledge of the medication. The bottom line: Only an experienced doctor should be prescribing methadone!

less than what has been prescribed unless advised by your prescriber. **Do not share your medications with anyone else or take someone else's; this is not only illegal, but also potentially lethal.** You are legally responsible for every pill that was prescribed to you. It is advisable for many reasons most notably your safety to receive prescriptions for pain medications from only ONE PRESCRIBER.

"Nontraditional" Medications For Cancer

As with any type of chronic pain, a multitude of medications can successfully be used to treat cancer-related pain. The following medications may all play a role in alleviating cancer-related pain, depending on the type of pain being treated. These "nontraditional" medications for pain have now in fact become the "gold standard" for treating certain types of pain. Most were initially developed for another purpose/condition, such as depression or seizure disorders, and have been found scientifically to help reduce pain independent of their intended effects. Often, these medications may be used alone or prescribed in combination with other types of pain medications, both traditional and nontraditional.

SOME ANTIDEPRESSANTS ARE POWERFUL PAIN RELIEVERS

The pain-relieving benefits of certain antidepressants have been proven for many years. Certain antidepressants are now actually FDA-approved for certain painful conditions, whereas others are used in an "off-label" fashion for pain control.

TCAs Should Be Used Cautiously

TCAs are medications such as amitriptyline, nortriptyline, imipramine, doxepin, and desipramine, which have been established as useful treatments for nerve injury (neuropathic) pain, headaches, and other pain syndromes. The most common side effects include constipation, dry mouth, blurred vision, tachycardia, and urinary retention. Use of these medications, especially amitriptyline, can be associated with causing serious heart rhythm abnormalities, so these medications need to be used cautiously in certain people.

Serotonergic Noradrenergic Reuptake Inhibitors (SNRIs) Are Widely Used for Chronic Pain

SNRIs are another group of antidepressants that have been shown to be effective for certain pain conditions, including cancer-related pain syndromes. Duloxetine (Cymbalta) is FDA-approved to treat painful diabetic neuropathy and fibromyalgia, and recently was shown to reduce chronic low back pain and osteoarthritis. Venlafaxaine (Effexor) is not FDA-approved for the treatment of pain, but some studies have shown it to be effective for the treatment of painful diabetic neuropathy, as well as chronic headaches. Minalcipran (Savella) is an FDA-approved medication for the treatment of fibromyalgia, and although it is used in other countries for the treatment of depression, it is not FDA-approved for this purpose. Desvenlafaxine (Pristiq) is a newly approved antidepressant, but formal studies regarding its efficacy in treating pain have not yet been published.

Serotonin-Specific Reuptake Inhibitors (SSRIs) Do Not Work Well for Pain

SSRIs such as fluoxetine (Prozac), citalopram (Celexa), escitalopram (Lexapro), and sertraline (Zoloft) have not been shown to be as effective as TCAs and SNRIs for pain reduction.

In addition, there is limited information to support the use of bupropion (Welbutrin), an antidepressant that does not "fit" into any of the other categories for the treatment of nerve injury (neuropathic) pain.

ANTISEIZURE MEDICATIONS VARY FOR CANCER PAIN

Antiseizure medications are commonly used for pain control, especially with neuropathic pain. One of the first such medications was carbamazepine (Tegretol). However, for the person with cancer-related pain, this medication has a somewhat limited role because it can cause bone marrow suppression. This is a potentially very serious side effect for someone with cancer who may already be taking chemotherapeutic medications that can do the same thing. Other antiseizure medications with FDA approval for a painful condition include gabapentin (Neurontin) and

Managing Opioid-Induced Constipation

These recommendations should be started on the first day you take any opioid drug, before constipation starts:

- Drink plenty of water.
- Follow a diet high in fiber.
- Be as active as you can.
- Use a stool softener or enema as directed by your health care provider.

Some Opioids Not Recommended for Cancer Pain

Demerol (Meperidine) Demerol is not a recommended drug to treat cancer pain because as it is metabolized in the body into a chemical that is toxic to the nervous system, which can lead to severe seizures and other adverse consequences.

Talwin, Stadol, Nubain These three opioid drugs—pentazocine (Talwin), butorphanol (Stadol), and nalbuphine (Nubain)—are not recommended for cancer-related pain because they all are designed to both activate and block the actions of opioid analgesics, which may result in unintentional withdrawal effects, such as delusions and hallucinations, as well as worsening pain.

141

What's New: Drugs That Can Treat Opioid-Induced Constipation

I've tried to drink water, eat fiber, and stay active, but the constipation continues. Is there anything else I can do? You might try a new type of medicine called *peripheral opioid antagonists*, which block the effect of opioids in the peripheral nervous system, where opioids are likely to cause constipation.

One such agent, Relistor (methylnaltrexone) must be injected in order to use it. This is approved for use by the FDA only in patients with terminal illness. Another agent, Entereg (alvimopan), is FDA-approved only for patients who need faster recovery following gastrointestinal surgeries (colon for example), must be administered in the hospital, and can only be used for 15 doses.

The drugs do not impede opioid action in the central nervous system, where they are likely to cause analgesia.

pregabalin (Lyrica). Specific studies have shown that combining gabapentin with an opioid may be better than using either medication alone for controlling pain.

Antiseizure medications that do not have FDA approval for the treatment of pain and have a lower likelihood of relieving cancer-related pain include lamotrigine (Lamictal), oxcarbazepine (Trileptal), and phenytoin (Dilantin).

Side effects of antiseizure medications vary from medication to medication (see the "Antiseizure Medication Side Effects" sidebar on p. 144).

LOCAL ANESTHETIC MEDICATIONS WORK FOR NERVE INJURY

Local anesthetic medications such as oral mexiletene or the topical lidocaine patch (Lidoderm) may be considered, especially for pain associated with nerve injury (neuropathic). Some doctors have used the lidocaine patch to treat bone-related cancer pain as well.

It's important to understand that these two medications are very different. The lidocaine patch is considered a topical drug because it acts locally under the patch on nerves or soft tissues that are causing local pain, and hence is a very safe medication. On the other hand, mexiletine is taken as a pill and is delivered through your bloodstream. At doses that may help to reduce pain, it commonly causes side effects, especially diarrhea and other gastrointestinal adverse effects.

STEROIDS ARE GOOD FOR BONE PAIN

Corticosteroids (e.g., steroids, prednisone, methylprednisolone, and dexamethasone) may be especially useful for cancer-related pain associated with bony involvement, especially when used in combination with other treatments. Some doctors suggest using high doses of steroids for short periods of time for many different types of severe cancer-related pain. Side effects include psychosis, depression, high blood sugar, muscle weakness, necrosis of certain bones, and reduced function of the immune system. In general, the likelihood of significant adverse effects increases the longer the medication is used.

BISPHOSPHONATES FOR METASTATIC BONE PAIN

Certain medications have been used for treatment of metastatic bone pain. Medications in this category include pamidronate (Aredia), zoledronic acid (Zometa), and ibandronate (Boniva). Although these may be helpful medications, there are reports of significant side effects including severe bone, joint, and muscle pain, as well as a risk of developing necrosis of the bone. Therefore, if a doctor recommends bisphosphonates, you need to discuss these possible side effects and how your doctor will monitor you for them.

OTHER TYPES OF MEDICATIONS FOR CANCER PAIN

The following nontraditional pain relievers are most often used when other approaches to pain reduction have not been successful, since use of these medications may be associated with abnormal or psychotic behavior:

- Baclofen, a medication usually prescribed to reduce muscle spasticity. Side effects include sedation and withdrawal symptoms such as seizures if the medication is stopped suddenly.
- Clonidine, FDA-approved for pain reduction when given epidurally. It is usually used for hypertension management when given by mouth or through a skin patch. Clonidine use is associated with a reduction in blood pressure and difficulty thinking.
- Stimulants such as methylphenidate, which may cause insomnia, nausea, or nervousness.
- Ketamine, an anesthetic that blocks a receptor in the nervous system known as the NMDA receptor, an action that has been shown to be effective for difficult-to-control cancer-associated pain. This drug is very powerful and should only be used by trained physicians.
- Dextromethorphan (the DM in cough syrups!). This also has a similar action as ketamine and is sometimes helpful to people with severe cancer-associated pain.
- Methadone, an opioid pain reliever that also has some activity on the NMDA receptor, which may help where nerve pain is part of the problem.

Antidepressants to Be Considered for Pain Control

Tricyclics
- Amitripityline (Elavil)
- Nortriptyline (Pamelor)
- Doxepin (Sinequan)
- Imirpramine (Tofranil)
- Desipramine (Norpramin)

SNRIs
- Duloxetine (Cymbalta)
- Venlafaxine (Effexor)
- Minalcipran (Savella)

Other
- Bupropion (Wellbutrin)

143

Antiseizure Medication Side Effects

Gabapentin (Neurontin): somnolence, dizziness, unsteadiness, weight gain, swelling of the lower extremities

Pregabalin (Lyrica): somnolence, dizziness, unsteadiness, weight gain, swelling of the lower extremities

Carbamazepine (Tegretol): bone marrow suppression, dizziness, difficulty thinking, visual changes

Topiramate (Topamax): sedation, visual changes, tingling in the extremities, weight loss

Divalproex sodium (Depakote): dizziness, weight gain, tremors, hair loss, liver toxicity

Lamotrigine (Lamictal): dizziness, double vision, headaches, severe rash

Oxcarbazepine (Trileptal): sedation, dizziness, nausea, headache, low serum sodium levels

Phenytoin (Dilantin): sedation, eye movement abnormalities, loss of balance, impaired absorption of vitamin D

Nonmedication Treatments for Cancer Pain

Certainly, doctors can treat cancer-associated pain by other means besides the use of medications. The following physical, psychological, and invasive treatments may be useful in alleviating the generalized weakness and pain of cancer.

PASSIVE PHYSICAL THERAPIES RELIEVE MUSCULOSKELETAL PAIN

Put Your Pain on Ice

Cold therapy can reduce swelling and provide pain relief for several hours. One can apply ice or cold packs to affected areas for fifteen minutes at a time. However, cold or ice packs need to be used very carefully on individuals who also have peripheral vascular disease and who have experienced tissue damage due to radiation therapy.

Therapeutic Massage Provides Temporary Relief

Therapeutic massage can help a wide variety of painful conditions, but tumors should not be aggressively massaged. It has been well established that massage therapy can provide almost immediate reduction of pain; however, equally well known is that these benefits are not long-lasting! If you find that therapeutic massage is helpful, you should seriously look into a therapeutic exercise program to help maintain the benefits of massage.

Immobilize New Fractures

Unlike with any noncancer pain condition, immobilization may be useful in some rare instances of cancer-related pain. For instance, when a new fracture is restricting the affected limb or joint, immobilization may be helpful in decreasing pain. The caveat here is to balance the benefit with the risk of developing additional pain as a consequence of the immobilization. Thus, if your doctor recommends immobilization, be sure to start moving the body part as soon as it is safe to do so. Prolonged, extended immobilization should always be avoided.

Transcutaneous Electrical Nerve Stimulation (TENS) Replaces Pain with Pleasant Tingling

A method of pain control, TENS is the application of a mild electrical current through the skin, resulting in a pleasant tingling sensation instead of pain. Although the mechanism of electrical stimulation is not 100 percent known, some doctors believe that stimulating touch and vibration nerves in the skin can block pain signals from that same area. Others believe that perhaps TENS increases the production of natural painkillers, called *endorphins*, in the body, resulting in pain reduction.

THERAPEUTIC EXERCISE CAN BE DONE AT HOME

For many patients with cancer-related pain, a therapeutic exercise program can have significant benefits, both on the pain and on the patient's functional abilities. Weak, tight muscles and stiff joints may respond well to a therapeutic exercise program. Although at times it is necessary for this to be completed through a formal PT program, many people can perform a therapeutic exercise program at home. If a person has significant functional limitations, a family member or a physical therapist can assist in the exercise program. Note that if bone fractures are suspected as a consequence of the cancer, weight-bearing exercises involving that bone need to be avoided.

RADIATION THERAPY HELPS PAINFUL METASTASES

Radiation therapy may be very useful for some patients with cancer-related pain. This has especially been shown for people with painful metastases to the bone. As with other treatments, the dose of radiation used needs to be carefully chosen by the radiation oncologist to provide the most benefit and the least adverse effects. Radiation therapy can be completed as well through intravenous injections.

Cancer Alert!

Not All PT Is Good and may be Bad for your Cancer

The following PT modalities that seem quite innocuous are actually not recommended for some people with cancer-related pain:

Heat (heating pad, hydrotherapy): Do not use heat on areas that have been recently treated with radiation therapy.

Ultrasound: This is not recommended over areas where a tumor is located.

ACUPUNCTURE RESTORES VITAL ENERGY FLOW

Acupuncture involves the placement of very small needles into the skin at points that have been shown to be associated with pain relief when they are stimulated. Acupuncture has been used for thousands of years and is associated with vital energy flow. It can be done with or without electrical stimulation.

PSYCHOLOGICAL THERAPIES PROVIDE COPING SKILLS

Psychological treatments to reduce pain are an important component of a comprehensive approach to pain management. These help the person with cancer-related pain develop coping skills as well as a sense of control over his or her cancer and the pain. To help alleviate pain, a pain psychologist should teach the patient techniques to help him or her self-treat the pain with "brain tricks."

Relaxation Helps Manage Stress

Often, simple relaxation techniques can be of great benefit to patients with cancer-related pain. Just learning how to reduce your stress reaction (see chapter 17) can have profound effects on reducing pain.

Hypnosis, Biofeedback, and Cognitive Distraction

Similarly, medical hypnosis and biofeedback training can also be used to provide significant degrees of pain relief. Cognitive distraction and reframing refers to techniques that guide people with cancer-related pain to focus on matters other than the pain.

Psychotherapy and Support Groups

Traditional psychotherapy may be helpful for patients who have developed significant depression and/or anxiety. Lastly, many cancer-related pain patients find that participation in a support group in their community can be very helpful.

INVASIVE TREATMENTS REMOVE OR DESTROY THE PAIN

Surgery to Remove the Painful Tumor

Surgery, either by curing the cancer through removal of the tumor or by removing part of the tumor that may be compressing a pain-sensitive structure, can be helpful for certain people with cancer-related pain.

Radiofrequency Ablation Destroys Pain

A technique known as *radiofrequency ablation* has been used to treat painful metastatic bone lesions to reduce pain. The radiofrequency technique uses heat generated from a radiofrequency machine to selectively destroy the pain nerves in the affected tissues.

Nerve Blocks Have Many Uses

Various types of nerve blocks (see chapter 9) may be considered for some patients with certain types of cancer-related pain. These can be:

- Diagnostic (to help diagnose the cause of the pain)
- Therapeutic (to treat/alleviate the pain)
- Prognostic (to help predict whether a particular procedure may provide long-lasting pain relief)
- Preemptive (to prevent pain associated with an operation or other type of procedure)

Medications from a Pump into your Spinal Fluid

Sometimes medication such as opioids can be directly infused into the spinal fluid regions by use of inserted devices or pumps. Medication pumps should be considered only after less-invasive approaches have failed.

Common Cancer Pain Syndromes

Associated with tumor:

- Spread of cancer (metastasis) to bones (skull, limbs, or spine)
- Metastasis to an organ of the body (liver, intestines, lung)
- Paraneoplastic syndrome (rare), an autoimmune disorder in which the body fights the wrong cells, resulting in a wide range of side effects such as blurred vision and difficulty swallowing

Associated with cancer treatment:

- Radiation treatment: intestinal inflammation, neuropathic pain, spinal cord injury, fibrotic changes
- Chemotherapy: joint pain, muscle pain, bone pain, abdominal pain, peripheral neuropathy-related pain, oral pain
- Pain following hormonal therapy: increased bone pain, joint pain, muscle pain
- Pain following surgical therapy: post-surgical pain, phantom pain, post-mastectomy pain, post-thoracotomy pain
- Pain following the use of bisphosphonate medications: increased bone pain

Neurolytic Procedures As a Last Resort

Rarely, in severe hard-to-treat circumstances, neurosurgeons may choose to actually destroy portions of the nervous system (neurolytic procedures) to reduce pain. This should be done only if the patient has fewer than three months to live, since after this period there is a chance that the pain will return, and when it does it is often much worse than it was before the procedure was done.

Diagnosing Cancer Pain

Poor treatment of cancer-related pain may result if the pain is not properly assessed. Remember that proper pain assessment is a two-way street. Both the patient and the doctor need to be actively involved and communicating with one another. The evaluation should occur when the pain is first experienced as well as at regular intervals after treatment is started. For ongoing treatment, it will be necessary to assess the response to therapy at regular intervals as well.

A physical examination including a neurological examination is necessary to help determine the cause of the pain. For example, specific abnormalities of neurological function noted on the examination may point to a nerve injury (neuropathic) source, which may then help the doctor pick the best treatments for this type of pain.

Needless to say—but perhaps it must be stated—identification of the cause of the pain is vital to its proper management. Common cancer-related pain syndromes are divided into those associated directly with the tumor and those associated with the cancer treatments (see the "Common Cancer Pain Syndromes" sidebar).

HELPFUL TESTS FOR CANCER PAIN

Often, your doctor will order a radiological test to see if your pain is caused by a spread of the cancer. Commonly ordered tests include MRI, CT scan, plain X-ray, bone scan, and diagnostic ultrasound.

Cancer Pain Explained

Although there are many different types of cancer-related pain, by definition cancer pain is any pain due to either direct invasion by the tumor into pain-sensitive structures or a complication of cancer therapy, such as from surgery, chemotherapy, or radiation. Keep in mind that processes unrelated to the cancer may also coexist for someone with cancer. For instance, a person with a life-long history of migraine headaches may still experience migraines even if he or she also has a cancer-related pain problem as well. The vast majority of people with severe cancer pain suffer from a syndrome that is due directly to the tumor itself. The most common cause of cancer-related pain is bone metastases, in other words when the cancer moves into the bone. Often, a person may experience more than one type of cancer-related pain, such as from direct tumor invasion and as the result of chemotherapy, and will also often have pain in more than one area of his or her body.

Metastasis of spine ▶

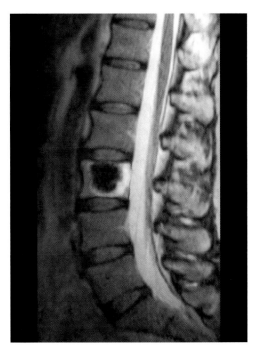

Examination Findings: Cancer Pain

Probably most critical to a
doctor's evaluation of cancer-
related pain is the patient's report
of the pain: what the pain feels
like, how severe it is, what makes
it better and what makes it worse,
the location of the pain, and its
pattern. The pattern of the pain
refers to features such as whether
it occurs on an intermittent or
continuous basis, predictably in
response to certain activities, or
in a random fashion. Once you
have initially assessed your pain,
you should share with your doctor
any change in the pain pattern or
any of its other features. It might
be useful for you or your family to
keep a pain diary to help everyone
involved get an accurate sense of
how the pain is affecting you.

The Natural Course of Cancer Pain

There is no singular natural course of cancer pain, as there are multiple types
and etiologies. For some, the pain will resolve as the cancer is controlled. Others,
however, may continue to experience cancer-related pain even after the cancer is
treated, because as in chemotherapy-related cancer pain, the pain may be caused
by injury to nerves associated with the cancer treatment.

CONCLUSION: MANY PAINS, MANY TREATMENTS

In summary, cancer-related pain comes in many forms. As such, many appropriate
treatment options exist, depending on the underlying cause of the pain. As with
other types of pain, no two patients may benefit from the same therapies. Thus,
it is important for you to find a doctor who is knowledgeable about evaluating all
types of cancer-related pain and who can find the best treatments for you.

Q & A *with*
Dr. Argoff and Dr. Galer

I have been treated successfully for breast cancer and am cured, according to my oncologist. I was given paclitaxel and my feet are burning and numb. My oncologist says I don't need to see him anymore. Who is going to treat my pain?

One of the consequences of improved treatment of cancer has been that more people than ever are successfully treated, while at the same time they are still experiencing cancer-related pain as the result of treatment side effects. In our experience, many oncologists do not continue to treat cancer-related pain because they feel the cancer has been cured. This places you in a precarious position. Our advice is for you to discuss this aspect of your care with your oncologist while you are still being treated for cancer; ask the oncologist what he or she will do if the cancer is cured but the pain persists. Will the oncologist continue to prescribe treatment? Will your primary care physician be expected to do so? Will the primary care physician refer you to a pain specialist? Plan ahead, by bringing this up with your oncologist.

I am being treated for metastatic prostate cancer to my spine. I am having side effects from the opioid medication I have been prescribed, particularly constipation. What can I do?

Very often, switching the opioid to a different one, a concept known as *opioid rotation*, can help reduce side effects but continue to provide pain relief. Different opioids attach to opioid receptors in our body uniquely from person to person, and thus what works best for one person may not work best for another person.

I cannot tolerate enough medication by mouth or through skin patches for my cancer pain. What can I do?

One option to consider is the use of medication directly administered into your spinal fluid (intrathecal space). Various types of medication—both opioid and nonopioid—can be delivered through this route. In general, this is more effective, with fewer side effects than through an oral, transdermal, intramuscular, or intravenous route. A test dose of medication would need to be completed, and then surgery to implant a medication delivery system that pumps the medication into your spinal fluid at prescribed doses. The pump needs to be refilled periodically, and the dose can be adjusted noninvasively through a special computer-based pump programmer.

151

PART 2

The Most Effective And Cutting-Edge Treatments For Pain

CHAPTER 8

Understanding Medications for Pain

Properly evaluate each drug's

benefit-to-risk ratio.

the PRESCRIPTION for CHRONIC PAIN MEDICINE

Although each pain condition may have particular medications that in general responds better than others, the same rules apply for picking first-line versus second-line and third-line drugs.

Try the ones with proven efficacy (i.e., pain-relieving abilities demonstrated in studies that compare the medication versus placebos) and with the least amount of potential side effects. Thus, just as the FDA evaluates drugs, you should always weigh a drug's benefits and risks for a so-called benefit:risk ratio, i.e., you need to find out if the chances are greater you will obtain more pain relief than side effect. Medications-for-pain can be divided into these categories:

- ✓ "Painkillers": anti-inflammatory drugs, nonsteroidal anti-inflammatory drugs (NSAIDs), cox-2 specific drugs, and acetaminophen
- ✓ Topical medicines
- ✓ Antiseizure medications
- ✓ Antidepressants
- ✓ Opioids (sometimes referred to as *narcotics*—because the term *narcotic* actually includes non-opioid medications that do not treat pain, we do not feel it is appropriate to use the term when describing an opioid drug)

The Golden Rule for Medication for Pain

A successful medication should reduce your pain with limited side effects, resulting in your ability to be more active. Put simply:

- If the good (pain relief) outweighs the bad (side effects) and you are noticing an improvement in your ability to participate in your normal daily activities, your current medication is a good fit for you.

- If the bad outweighs the good and you are not noticing a meaningful reduction in your pain at the highest tolerated dose, or if you are having bad side effects, your medication is not appropriate for you and should be discontinued (under supervision by your doctor).

Rules For Taking Medications, Part I

When taking medications for pain, there are a few simple rules to follow. Keeping these in mind will help you become a co-director in managing your medication regimen.

RULE 1: EVERY PERSON IN PAIN IS DIFFERENT

Just because your friend with the same pain condition gets good pain relief from a certain drug doesn't mean you will too. And even if the two of you experience relief from the same medication, the doses that deliver that relief may be very different. Also, one of you may experience side effects from a certain drug and the other may not.

RULE 2: ALWAYS CHANGE DOSES ONE DRUG AT A TIME

Your doctor should always start every medicine at the lowest possibly effective dose and gradually increase it by the lowest possible increment every three to seven days (depending on the medicine and how you are reacting to it with regard to the amount of pain relief and side effects you experience). Remember, your doctor should do this with only one drug at a time.

RULE 3: KEEP IN CLOSE CONTACT WITH YOUR DOCTOR WHEN ADJUSTING YOUR DOSES

When your doctor changes your medication, you should contact your doctor or his staff at least once per week until the dose is stable. If you ever have any questions, you should immediately call the doctor's office for answers.

RULE 4: YOU MUST BE AN ACTIVE PARTICIPANT IN YOUR TREATMENT

Trying to find the best pain relief with medicines (or any other treatments) requires that you take some responsibility. You must tell your doctor what changes have occurred with the medicine, good and bad, and follow his or her advice closely. If you have started a new medication for any medical condition—even an antibiotic for an infection—you should inform your doctor of this change because it may actually interfere with the pain treatment that your doctor has prescribed for you. By reading this book, you are learning how to best do this and are becoming your most important advocate!

WHAT IS "OFF-LABEL USE" OF PAIN MEDICATIONS?

Many, if not most, of the medications doctors (especially pain doctors) prescribe to their patients are off label, meaning the medication is being prescribed to treat a condition that has not been FDA-approved for that condition. You should realize that this practice is very common, and usually is based on your doctor's experience with the drug in similar patients and on his or her reading of studies in the medical journals showing good results with the drug for your condition.

Often, a drug company will not pursue FDA approval for a pain condition because either it is too costly or the drug's patent life will expire before the FDA will approve the new indication, and thus a generic copycat will be available before the company can obtain a return on its investment (the investment to obtain FDA approval for a drug is often more than tens of millions, even hundreds of millions of dollars). But your doctor should inform you when he or she is prescribing a medication off label and why he or she thinks it will help you. This is an absolutely allowed practice in the United States.

Frequently Asked Questions For Managing Pain

It is only natural to feel confused by the many facets of pain management—even for doctors, this is complicated stuff! In this section, we outline some of the most frequently asked questions on the topic of medication for pain.

WHAT MAKES A SUCCESSFUL MEDICATION FOR PAIN?

It is critical to have realistic expectations. Unfortunately, with one medication, most people with chronic pain do not experience a reduction in pain of greater than 50 percent, although it may be possible to experience near complete pain relief with the right mixture of medications at the right dose working with appropriate nonmedication treatments. Still, it is important to accept that, even with the best treatment, you will likely not achieve 100 percent relief from your chronic pain. "Success" in pain management is measured not only by the degree of pain relief, but also by achieving this relief without intolerable side effects, while increasing your ability to function and participate in desired activities.

⚡ Alert! Over the Counter (OTC) Doesn't Guarantee Safety

Just because a drug is available OTC without a prescription does not mean it is safe or has proven pain-relieving capabilities. Acetaminophen (Tylenol) has very serious potential side effects, such as liver toxicity, and oral NSAIDs (Motrin, Advil, ibuprofen, aspirin, Aleve, naproxen) can all cause very serious kidney abnormalities if not taken in proper doses. Also, most of the OTC pain creams/gels/patches (Bengay, Icy Hot) have little to no proven efficacy.

Names of NSAID Medications (Brand Names)

- Ibuprofen (Advil, Motrin)
- Naproxen (Aleve)
- Ketorolac (Toradol)
- Diclofenac (Voltaren, Pennsaid)
- Acetaminophen (Tylenol*) (In countries other than the United States, it is called Paracetamol.)

* Acetaminophen is not technically an NSAID, but for our purposes we'll put it here. Acetaminophen, like the NSAIDs, does inhibit cyclooxygenase (COX), an enzyme responsible for the production of prostaglandins, which are important mediators of inflammation and pain. However, acetaminophen has little true anti-inflammatory action and believe it or not, its true pain-relieving mechanism is still not known.

WHEN SHOULD YOU STOP TAKING A MEDICATION FOR PAIN?

You should stop taking a medication for pain if either of the following occurs:

- If after you achieve the highest-tolerated dose of a medication, the medication does not reduce your pain in a meaningful way, you should stop taking that medication. Although it's up to you to decide what constitutes "meaningful" pain reduction, studies suggest that most individuals with chronic pain feel that an approximately 30 percent reduction in pain is meaningful to them.
- You should stop taking a medication if it causes you bad side effects, even if it seems to effectively reduce your pain.

WHY SHOULD EVERY MEDICINE'S DOSE BE GRADUALLY INCREASED OR DECREASED?

In doctors' terms, the processes of increasing and decreasing a medication dose are known as *titration* and *tapering*, respectively. It is not known at which dose any medication for pain will work or cause side effects for any individual patient. As we mentioned earlier, every patient is different. Therefore, you will not be able to tell whether a medicine is the right one for you until it is titrated to the correct dose. Many people do not experience meaningful relief until they are taking the highest dose they can tolerate, meaning the largest dose they can comfortably take every day without experiencing bad side effects.

Also, very importantly, if you and your doctor agree that a certain medication for pain is not right for you and you both decide that you should be taken off the medication, you also need to decide how to stop it. Most often, it may be necessary to gradually reduce your dose. It may be dangerous and/or very unpleasant to stop taking certain medications such as opioids "cold turkey" because you may experience withdrawal symptoms (this does not mean you're "addicted!").

WHAT ABOUT POTENTIAL LONG-TERM EFFECTS OF DRUGS?

This is a very important question. When your doctor prescribes medication for the treatment of chronic pain, he or she should tell you about the potential side effects after long-term use. Unlike treating acute pain, where a medication is prescribed for only a short period of time, if a medication is successful in treating your chronic pain it will be prescribed for an indefinite period of time—months or even years.

In addition to side effects that you may notice immediately, you must also be aware of potential adverse effects that may develop slowly and that you may not notice right away. Therefore, when prescribing a medication for chronic pain, your doctor should explain to you any risks of taking that particular drug. Additionally, when taking a medication for a long period of time, it may be necessary for your doctor to screen you periodically for potential adverse effects associated with that drug, such as checking your liver or kidney function through blood tests as well as blood counts, depending on which drug you are taking.

Rules For Taking Medications, Part II

If you are not following any of these rules right now, you should discuss these issues with your doctor so that you and your pain can be better treated.

RULE 1: YOU HAVE TO GIVE THE MEDICATION A FAIR CHANCE TO WORK

Too often, people with chronic pain will stop taking a medication prematurely because they believe it doesn't work. What they don't realize is that if they had increased the dose gradually (under a doctor's supervision), they may have experienced excellent pain relief. You don't want to miss this potentially life-changing opportunity, do you?

RULE 2: EACH MEDICATION SHOULD BE TAKEN DAILY ON A REGULAR SCHEDULE

Most medication for chronic pain should be prescribed around the clock to ensure that a steady level of the drug is in your system at all times. You should be taking the medicine every day at the same time(s)—not based on when your pain is bad— to keep the same amount of the drug in your body. (There are some exceptions to this rule for specific types of medicine, which we describe later in this chapter.)

RULE 3: TRY TO MINIMIZE THE NUMBER OF DIFFERENT MEDICATIONS-FOR-PAIN THAT YOU ARE TAKING

You should always aim to take the least amount of medication possible. Remember what you just learned: You should continue taking a medication for pain only if it is giving you meaningful pain relief, with no or few side effects, and you are able to be more active. Many times, people stay on certain drugs seemingly forever, even when the drugs are not helping at all and should be stopped. All medication has potential side effects (and added costs!), so why take a drug if the benefit:risk ratio is not in your favor? You and your doctor should review every medication for pain you are taking at least every 3 months.

Names of FDA-Approved Topical Pain Drugs (Brand Names)

- Lidocaine patch 5% (Lidoderm): FDA-approved for the relief of pain associated with postherpetic neuralgia (PHN)

- Topical diclofenac sodium topical solution 1.5% (Pennsaid): FDA-approved to treat the signs and symptoms of OA of the knee

- Diclofenac sodium topical gel 1% (Voltaren Gel): FDA-approved for relief of the pain of OA of joints amenable to topical treatment, such as the knees and hands

- Diclofenac epolamine topical patch (Flector): FDA-approved for the topical treatment of acute pain due to minor strains, sprains, and contusions

159

Alert! Compounded Topical Drugs: Beware!

A compounding pharmacy is a type of pharmacy that will prepare a specialized medication to fill an individual patient prescription authorized by a doctor. Although compounding pharmacies are legal, they are not regulated by the FDA with respect to quality control. Compounding pharmacies use their own homegrown, poorly studied (and usually not studied at all!) concoctions that have not been evaluated by the FDA. The topical drugs that a compounding pharmacy may make for you have not been properly tested, and therefore:

- May not even penetrate the skin, and thus have no real effect on your pain
- May cause too much of the drug to penetrate the skin and get too much into the bloodstream, potentially causing serious side effects
- May cause severe skin reactions and allergies
- May interact negatively with its packaging and result in the absorption of potentially toxic compounds

Commonly Used Medications For Pain

The NSAIDs are a first-line therapy for many chronic pain states, such as arthritis pain and certain types of headaches. However, in other states, such as chronic myofascial pain, neuropathic pain, and fibromyalgia, in which there is no significant degree of active inflammation, these drugs less commonly produce significant amounts of pain relief.

NSAIDS

As the name implies, NSAIDs act by reducing the inflammatory response. Some recent studies have suggested that some of these drugs may produce pain relief by having a direct effect in the nervous system, independent of their anti-inflammatory activities.

POTENTIAL ADVERSE EFFECTS ASSOCIATED WITH NSAIDS

Acute
- Nausea and stomach upset (except acetaminophen)

Long-term
- Liver abnormalities
- Kidney abnormalities
- Stomach or intestinal ulcers (does not generally apply to acetaminophen)
- Cardiovascular adverse events (heart attack, stroke, high blood pressure)
- New data is emerging that indicates chronic use can increase the risk of cardiovascular problems.
- If migraine patients take these drugs too often (daily or near daily), they may cause a daily headache syndrome called *rebound headache*.

COX-2 INHIBITOR ANTI-INFLAMMATORY DRUGS

COX-2 inhibitors work on pain by decreasing the amount of inflammation at the site of injury, the same mechanism with which the traditional NSAIDs work. However, unlike the traditional NSAIDs, these drugs were designed in the laboratory to specifically interact with only the inflammation chemicals at the site of injury, and not to have any activity on similar chemicals that are also present elsewhere in the body, such as in the stomach. Thus, pharmaceutical companies designed these drugs in hopes of keeping the good and eliminating the bad effects of NSAIDs. Most of these drugs, like the NSAIDs, have also been shown to potentially increase the risk of cardiovascular adverse events.

These drugs have been shown to relieve pain associated with both rheumatoid arthritis (RA) and osteoarthritis (OA) pain, as well as treating acute pain from migraine headaches, tension-type headaches, and some musculoskeletal pain conditions, such as sprains and strains.

It is important to realize that COX-2 drugs have never been shown in studies to relieve pain better than NSAIDs. However, some pain sufferers do report that they feel COX-2 drugs give them better pain relief than NSAIDs.

THE COX-2 LANDSCAPE AFTER VIOXX

Many of you may remember the media attention given to COX-2 inhibitors during their introduction and FDA hearings. In the late 1990s, we remember the full-blown cover stories in *Time* and *Newsweek* proclaiming them as "super aspirins" that would cure all pains without the side effects commonly associated with NSAIDs, such as gastritis and stomach ulcers, even when the studies showed that their pain relief wasn't any better than that provided by ibuprofen (Motrin and Advil).

In 1999, both Celebrex and Vioxx were introduced to the U.S. market and rapidly became the most frequently prescribed new drugs in the United States, with sales in the United States exceeding $3 billion in 2000 and more than 100 million prescriptions written that year. In 2001, Pfizer's sales of Celebrex alone amounted to $3.1 billion. Then suddenly, on September 27, 2004, Merck voluntarily took Vioxx (rofecoxib) off the market, due to studies suggesting an increased risk of heart attack and stroke.

In February 2005, the FDA Arthritis Drug Advisory Committee had several days of hearings on COX-2 inhibitors, evaluating studies of Celebrex, Bextra, and Vioxx. They concluded unanimously that all three of these drugs did increase the risk of heart attack and stroke, and recommended that the strongest possible warnings—so-called *Black-box Warnings*—be placed on the drugs' bottle or box to notify patients of these potential serious dangers. When the FDA asked the panel if each of the drugs should be banned, they voted 31 to 1 against banning Celebrex, 17 to 13 against banning Bextra, and 17 to 15 against banning Vioxx. The panelists of doctors and researchers believed that for some patients the benefits outweighed the risks, as long as both the prescribing doctor and the patient were made aware of the data.

In April 2005, Pfizer removed Bextra from the market. Today, in the United States only one COX-2 inhibitor is still on the market: Celebrex. Arcoxia, another Merck COX-2 inhibitor, is currently sold in Europe, Asia, and South America.

Names of COX-2 Medications (Brand Names)

- Celecoxib (Celebrex)
- Rofecoxib (Vioxx): The manufacturer of Vioxx removed the drug from the market in 2005 because it caused an increased risk of cardiovascular adverse events (heart attack and stroke).
- Valdecoxib (Bextra): The FDA removed Bextra from the market in 2005 because it caused an increased risk of cardiovascular adverse events (heart attack and stroke).
- Etoricoxib (Arcoxia): This drug is not approved in the United States, but it is available in Europe, Asia, and Latin America.

161

What's New: Lidocaine Patch 5% (Lidoderm)

Though other topical lidocaine formulations are available (and other topical novocaine-like drugs), Lidoderm is the only currently available local anesthetic drug formulation that causes pain relief (analgesia) without causing skin numbness (anesthesia). It is approved by the FDA to treat the chronic nerve pain of PHN. Clinical studies have also reported that it can also provide pain relief in other pain conditions, such as diabetic neuropathy pain, carpal tunnel syndrome, OA pain, and low back pain, although these uses are not FDA-approved.

Because its formulation is so unique, it should not be substituted for other topical lidocaine products. Many doctors and insurance companies do not understand this major difference, which has a significant effect on treatment efficacy.

How does it work? The lidocaine from the patch continually penetrates the skin and finds its way to the abnormal pain nerves under the skin that are causing electrical pain signals. When pain nerves get damaged or inflamed, they cause pain signals to go into the spinal cord and brain, even when there is no reason to. When lidocaine interacts with damaged or inflamed nerves, it quiets them down, resulting in fewer pain signals being sent to your brain.

Topical Analgesics Reduce Side Effects

With the proper formulation (special ingredients to help the drug penetrate the skin), topical drugs can be excellent chronic pain medications for when the pain is coming from muscles, nerves, or joints. And because extremely little of the drug gets into the bloodstream, it is less common than with oral analgesics that serious side effects occur. As you would expect, the most likely side effects are skin reactions such as rashes, but these are not very common. Also, because little gets into the blood, there is very little chance of drug-to-drug interactions.

HOW DOES A TOPICAL DRUG DIFFER FROM A TRANSDERMAL DRUG?

A lot of doctors and pharmacists still don't understand the critically important distinctions between topical and transdermal drug formulations. Like topical drugs, transdermal drugs are also applied to the skin, usually in a patch (Duragesic fentanyl pain patch, nicotine patch, estrogen patch, topical nitrates, etc.), though they can also be in a gel (testosterone gel). However, unlike topical drugs, transdermal drugs must result in the drug getting into the blood in significant amounts, since the drug doesn't work locally. For pain relief the drug must enter the brain, spinal cord, or organs to work. Therefore, the side effects of transdermal drugs are the same as those you can expect when taking the drug by mouth or injection since similar amounts of the medication enter the bloodstream.

Topical NSAIDS Are First-Line Treatments

The recently FDA-approved topical NSAIDs are now first-line pain treatments for OA and sports injury pains (sprains, strains, and contusions). Although other topical NSAIDs have been available in other parts of the world, such as Europe, Asia, and Latin America, these formulations have little proven efficacy.

TOPICAL NSAIDS (BRAND NAME)

- Topical diclofenac solution 1.5% (Pennsaid): FDA-approved for the signs and symptoms of OA of the knee
- Diclofenac topical gel 1% (Voltaren Gel): approved for the pain of OA of joints amenable to topical treatment, such as those of the knees and hands
- Diclofenac epolamine topical patch 1.3% (Flector Patch): approved for minor sports injury pain

TOPICAL NSAID SIDE EFFECTS

- Acute: skin rash
- Chronic: minimal risk of gastrointestinal, renal, kidney, and cardio-vascular problems
- The oral form has been associated rarely with liver abnormalities that most often self-resolve. This finding has also extremely rarely been reported in patients taking some topical diclofenac products; recently an FDA warning has been issued regarding the possibility of liver function abnormalities with use of Voltaren 1% gel. If you are prescribed the Voltaren 1% gel, be sure to ask your doctor to arrange for you to have blood tests done to check your liver function within 4 to 8 weeks of starting it. It may be that all drugs with the medication diclofenac present a risk for this adverse event.

Antiseizure Medications (Neuromodulators)

For more than fifty years, drugs that have been used primarily to treat seizures (epilepsy) have also been used to treat certain types of chronic pain, such as neuropathic pain and migraines. In fact, since the mid–1990s, two of these seizure drugs (gabapentin and pregabalin) have become first-line treatments for many nerve pain (neuropathic pain) conditions. To lessen confusion among patients and doctors, some of these drugs are now also referred to as *neuromodulators*.

All of the antiseizure drugs are thought to reduce nerve pain by quieting the abnormal nerves that are signaling "pain" in the central nervous system, brain, and spinal cord. However, the way each antiseizure drug reduces these abnormal signals differs, since many of these drugs interact with different brain and spinal cord chemicals. It is still not known exactly how some of these medications work to alleviate pain.

ANTISEIZURE MEDS HELP WITH NERVE PAIN

Antiseizure medications have been used to treat chronic nerve pain for several decades. It was originally thought that these drugs could help only with sharp, shooting, electric-like types of nerve pain. However, current research suggests that in many patients with nerve pain, these drugs can help with other types of pain qualities, including constant, dull, aching, or burning pain.

What's New: Topical Diclofenac for OA: Pennsaid versus Voltaren Gel

It is important to recognize the different approved indicated uses of these drugs:

- Topical diclofenac sodium topical solution 1.5% (Pennsaid) is FDA-approved to treat the signs and symptoms of OA of the knee, meaning it has been proven to improve knee pain, physical function (your ability to do things), and overall well-being.
- Diclofenac sodium topical gel 1% (Voltaren Gel) is FDA-approved for the relief of pain of OA of the joints amenable to topical treatment, such as the knees and hands; it's been proven only to improve the pain associated with OA.
- Voltaren Gel failed to show an improvement of function and overall health in OA patients, whereas Pennsaid did prove that it relieves the pain of knee OA and improves function and overall health. Moreover, Pennsaid has demonstrated it relieves OA pain equally as well as an oral NSAID with fewer side effects, but Voltaren Gel has never been studied head-to-head with an oral NSAID.

(Disclaimer: Dr. Galer helped develop Pennsaid and his current employer helps market the drug.)

163

Alert! Side Effects Associated with Antiseizure Medications

Drug	Acute	Chronic
All	Dizziness Sedation/fatigue Memory/thinking difficulty	
Gabapentin (Neurontin)	Peripheral edema (swelling of feet, legs)	None currently known
Pregabalin (Lyrica)	Peripheral edema	None currently known
Topiramate (Topamax)	Tingling feelings Loss of appetite	None currently known
Phenytoin (Dilantin)	Rare, possibly fatal, skin rash (Stevens-Johnson Syndrome)	Gingival hyperplasia (abnormal growth of gingiva in the mouth)
Carbamazepine (Tegretol)	Rare liver toxicity	Bone marrow suppression (rare) Liver toxicity (rare) —Note that blood needs to be checked regularly for blood count and liver function tests when taking carbamazepine
Valproic acid (Depakote)	Weight gain Hair loss Liver toxicity	Liver toxicity (blood needs to be checked regularly for liver function tests) Weight gain
Lamotrigine (Lamictal)	Stevens-Johnson Syndrome	Stevens-Johnson Syndrome
Oxcarbazepine (Trileptal)	None currently known	None currently known

The antiseizure drugs with the strongest evidence for efficacy in neuropathic pain conditions (e.g., PHN and painful diabetic peripheral neuropathy) are:

- Gabapentin (Neurontin): FDA-approved to treat PHN
- Pregabalin (Lyrica): FDA-approved to treat PHN and painful diabetic neuropathy
- Carbamazepine (Tegretol): FDA-approved to treat trigeminal neuralgia. Note that we haven't mentioned this drug in the Neuropathic Pain chapter because it should not be used for PHN, diabetic neuropathy, or RSD/CRPS. Because of its potential serious side effects, it should only be used first line to treat another uncommon nerve pain condition of the face called trigeminal neuralgia, where it works very reliably.

CHRONIC MIGRAINES CAN BE RELIEVED

Growing scientific evidence also suggests that some antiseizure drugs, when taken daily, can help reduce the frequency of chronic migraines. The antiseizure drugs that have the strongest evidence for efficacy in treating chronic migraines are:

- Topiramate (Topamax): FDA-approved to prevent the occurrence of chronic migraines
- Valproic acid (Depakote): FDA-approved to prevent the occurrence of chronic migraines
- Gabapentin (Neurontin): not FDA-approved, but several studies have demonstrated efficacy

Antidepressants Even If You're Not Blue

Antidepressants have been used to treat many different types of chronic pain for several decades. It is important to realize that these medications can be helpful in alleviating pain even if you are not depressed.

Two different types of antidepressant drugs are used to treat pain, and each works on different brain and spinal cord chemicals: tricyclic antidepressants (TCAs) and serotonergic noradrenergic reuptake inhibitors (SNRIs); see sidebar for examples of these medications. Another class of antidepressants, the serotonin-specific reuptake inhibitors (SSRIs), is sometimes used, but studies have not demonstrated that these drugs have major pain-relieving capabilities.

All of these drugs were first studied and used to treat depression, which is why they are still called *antidepressants*. When these drugs were initially discovered, doctors were unaware of their potential to help treat pain. In this section, we will outline the various types of antidepressant medications, as well as how they may be used to help treat your chronic pain.

Types of Antiseizure Drugs (Brand Names)

Pregabalin (Lyrica)
Gabapentin (Neurontin)
Topiramate (Topamax)
Phenytoin (Dilantin)
Carbamazepine (Tegretol)
Oxcarbazepine (Trileptal)
Valproic acid (Depakote)
Lamotrigine (Lamictal)

165

ACUTE SIDE EFFECTS ASSOCIATED WITH TCAS

- Anxiety/restlessness
- Confusion/poor memory
- Constipation
- Dizziness
- Drowsiness/fatigue
- Dry mouth
- Impaired vision
- Irregular heart rhythm*
- Nausea/loss of appetite/upset stomach
- Orthostatic hypotension (blood pressure falls with standing)*
- Sexual dysfunction
- Shaking
- Increased sweating
- Urinary retention
- Weight gain

* These side effects are rare, but they can lead to very serious consequences if they occur. Therefore, your doctor should check your blood pressure and EKG prior to prescribing a TCA drug and also while you are on this type of medication.

Though TCAs are commonly used to treat many chronic pain syndromes, a lot of patients—especially the elderly—cannot tolerate the side effects of these drugs. Thus, despite the potential benefit of these drugs, their side effects outweigh any pain-relieving effects they might provide. But, if other types of pain-relieving drugs are not working then the TCAs should still be tried.

TCAS WORK

Doctors prescribe TCAs because they can be excellent pain relievers for people in many chronic pain states. Clinical studies have demonstrated that TCAs can relieve the pain of peripheral neuropathy (such as diabetic neuropathy), PHN, chronic low back pain, chronic migraine headaches, and chronic tension-type headaches.

It's important to note that these drugs often produce significant pain relief quicker and at much lower doses than are needed to treat depression. For instance, nortriptyline needs to be given at 150 mg per day for at least four weeks before it begins to relieve depression, whereas to treat migraines, tension-type headaches, or neuropathic pain the average dose is 10–50 mg per day, and its pain-relieving effect may occur within one week once the correct dose is found for a patient.

Chronic-pain patients and their doctors should also realize that different TCAs can affect the same person in distinct ways (both good and bad). Therefore, if you are not getting sufficient pain relief or if you are experiencing bad side effects from one TCA drug, that doesn't mean all TCAs will have the same effect on you. Because all the TCAs differ dramatically in how they affect the chemicals in your brain and spinal cord, you should try several TCA drugs before you give up on the possibility that these drugs might be of benefit to you.

SSRIS DO NOT WORK WELL FOR PAIN

Unlike TCAs, most studies have shown that SSRIs do not relieve most pain conditions. In fact, except for their potential use in chronic migraine and chronic tension-type headache, these drugs are not considered good pain drugs as they have shown little to no pain-relieving abilities.

SSRIs are a class of medication widely prescribed to treat depression and anxiety. Thus, if you are depressed or you have an anxiety disorder (both of which are common in chronic pain patients due to their pain) these drugs may be a good choice for you, but to treat your psychological disorder, not to treat your pain.

SEROTONERGIC AND NORADRENERGIC REUPTAKE INHIBITORS (SNRIS)

Clinical study evidence strongly suggests that the SNRI duloxetine (Cymbalta) can relieve several types of chronic pain, including neuropathic pain, fibromyalgia, OA pain, and chronic low back pain. In fact, duloxetine has FDA approval for use in treating diabetic peripheral neuropathic pain (DPNP) and fibromyalgia, and at the time of this writing it is under FDA review for a general chronic pain indication. Another SNRI, venlafaxine (Effexor), has some studies showing pain relief for the treatment of OA and some neuropathic pain. These drugs are also FDA-approved to treat depression and generalized anxiety disorder.

Classes of Antidepressant Medications

TCAs
- Amitriptyline (Elavil)
- Nortriptyline (Pamelor)
- Desipramine (Norpramin)
- Doxepin (Sinequan)
- Imipramine (Tofranil)

SNRIs
- Venlafaxine (Effexor)
- Duloxetine (Cymbalta)
- Desvenlafaxine (Pristiq)

SSRIs (not recommended to treat chronic pain)
- Fluoxetine (Prozac)
- Paroxetine (Paxil)
- Sertraline (Zoloft)
- Citalopram (Celexa)
- Escitalopram (Lexapro)

167

What's New: Duloxetine for the Management of Chronic Pain

Although the efficacy of duloxetine (Cymbalta) in managing diabetic painful neuropathy (DPN) has been established for some time, long-term data has been lacking. However, recent evidence suggests that the drug can alleviate the pain associated with DPN for more than six months. This is good news for patients with DPN who are looking for a "maintenance" medication.

Can duloxetine be used to treat other types of pain? Recently, convincing evidence shows that, in addition to treating DPN, duloxetine can improve pain and associated symptoms in patients with various arthritic conditions, chronic low back pain, and fibromyalgia. That is why the FDA is currently reviewing all the scientific study data to determine whether it should grant duloxetine a general "chronic pain" indication.

Tizanidine (Zanaflex) for Tension-Type Headache

Tizanidine is a fairly unique drug in that it acts on alpha-2-adrenergic receptors, a neurotransmitter system in the nerves and muscles, and is considered a "muscle relaxant" type of drug. However, like many pain-relieving medications, the specific mechanism by which this drug relieves pain is not known.

Studies have shown that tizanidine can reduce tension-type headaches in some patients. Other studies have shown that it also might work to alleviate pain in some people with acute back pain or musculoskeletal pain.

Based on these studies and clinical experience, we think tizanidine can be a good medication for the treatment of tension-type headaches and perhaps for patients with some muscle pains. However, many patients experience more side effects than pain relief from tizanidine. See Table 8.2.

Table 8.2: Acute and Chronic Side Effects Associated with Tizanidine

Acute	• Sedation • Dry mouth • Decrease in blood pressure (uncommon)
Chronic	• Fatigue • Increased liver enzymes (very uncommon)

Systemic Local Anesthetic Drugs

Systemic local anesthetic drugs, such as an intravenous lidocaine infusion and oral mexiletine, work in neuropathic pain therapy by quieting the abnormal pain signals being generated in injured nerves, in both the central nervous system (brain and spinal cord) as well as the peripheral nerves. Due to the potential serious side effects associated with these drugs, they are generally prescribed only by pain specialists.

THE TWO TYPES OF SYSTEMIC LOCAL ANESTHETIC DRUGS (ROUTE OF ADMINISTRATION)

- Lidocaine (Intravenous Infusion): With intravenous lidocaine infusion, a doctor inserts an intravenous line into your arm and lidocaine slowly drips into your vein until a small amount is in your body, relieving your pain. Most commonly, this procedure takes place in a specialized pain clinic and may take several hours from start to finish.
- Mexiletine (pill): This oral tablet drug is FDA-approved to treat irregular heart rhythms, but it has been shown in some studies to relieve nerve pain for some patients.

Very good evidence suggests that an intravenous lidocaine infusion can significantly reduce many types of nerve injury pain, and also perhaps migraines. However, the problem with intravenous lidocaine infusions is that they provide most patients with only a few hours of pain relief. Rarely, though, some patients can experience days or even weeks of relief after one treatment. Studies have also shown that taking mexiletine (an oral pill) can also alleviate nerve pain, though many patients often experience intolerable side effects, most commonly nausea.

Systemic versus Topical Lidocaine

Lidocaine is a drug that pain specialists use both as an intravenous injection and as a daily topical patch. Both ways of administering lidocaine have been shown to alleviate certain types of pains. However, injecting lidocaine into the bloodstream via an infusion ("systemic" administration) has a lot more potential side effects.

Systemic drugs work by entering the bloodstream and traveling throughout the body. Thus, all drugs taken orally (pills, capsules, tablets, etc.) are systemic drugs. All drugs given intravenously are systemic drugs. Many medications in a patch are also systemic (called *transdermal*), including fentanyl and hormones.

Acute Side Effects Associated with SSRIs

- Anhedonia (inability to experience pleasure from normal activities)
- Anxiety/restlessness
- Diarrhea
- Dizziness
- Drowsiness/impaired sleep
- Headache or exacerbation of headache
- Nausea/loss of appetite/upset stomach
- Sexual dysfunction
- Shaking
- Urinary retention
- Weight gain

169

Medication Alert!

Acute Side Effects of Systemic Local Anesthetics

Intravenous lidocaine infusion

- Dizziness
- Ringing in ears
- Irregular heart rhythm (this rarely occurs, because the treatment is given under a doctor's supervision and the drug is very slowly dripped into the bloodstream)

Mexiletine

- Nausea (this can be lessened by taking the drug with food)
- Diarrhea
- Dizziness
- Anxiety (in patients with a history of anxiety disorder)
- Irregular heart rhythm (this should rarely occur since the drug's dose should be very slowly increased and pain relief typically occurs at doses far below that which can affect the heart)

This differs from topical therapies that utilize the active medication formulated for topical delivery (e.g., Lidoderm [lidocaine patch 5%] and topical NSAIDs). These work locally in the skin, muscles, and peripheral nerves where the drug is applied. Very little amounts of the drug actually get into the bloodstream and thus overall are much safer than systemic drugs.

IV lidocaine infusion has mostly only been shown to work on neuropathic pain conditions, whereas the lidocaine patch has been shown to help patients with not only peripheral neuropathic pain but also OA, back pain, and other local pain conditions.

Steroids Greatly Reduce Inflammation But Have Issues

Steroids are strong anti-inflammatory agents. Contrary to what some people believe, steroids are not pain relievers in the true sense; they have no direct mechanism for reducing pain. However, for a tiny percentage of chronic pain patients, steroids may be useful. When other drugs do not work, steroids can be given successfully in a pulsed oral dose (a high dose with a quick taper) for certain conditions, such as acute, difficult-to-treat migraines and during the early stages of Reflex Sympathetic Dystrophy (also known as *Complex Regional Pain Syndrome*). These drugs are also sometimes prescribed for certain types of chronic arthritis (including OA) and as interventional nerve block treatment for back pain.

SIDE EFFECTS ASSOCIATED WITH STEROIDS

Acute	Chronic
• Euphoria	• Ulcer
• Gastrointestinal (e.g., nausea)	• Osteoporosis
• Weight gain	• Physical dependence (the steroid dose must be slowly decreased; if stopped suddenly, it could cause serious medical problems)
	• Weight gain

Sedative/Hypnotic Drugs Don't Kill Pain

As the name implies, these drugs cause you to feel sedated and have a "hypnotiz-ing" effect. In other words, they make you feel tired and more relaxed, but they offer no true pain-relieving mechanism. In the past, sedative/hypnotic medica-tions were sometimes used to treat chronic pain, despite a lack of evidence for their efficacy. Luckily, today these drugs are being prescribed less and less frequently for pain disorders. However, unfortunately, some doctors still prescribe sedatives/hypnotics, so it is important for you to learn about these medications and avoid them.

Although sedatives/hypnotics may make you feel less bothered by your pain, more often they cause people to fall asleep. Additionally, these drugs can cause cognitive impairment (e.g., memory and concentration deficits) and can lead to a number of chronic side effects, including a potential for both a physical depen-dence and an addiction. Briefly, physical dependence means that after taking a drug chronically for months, you may develop withdrawal symptoms if you stop the drug suddenly; addiction is when you lose control over taking the medication and you start to take the medication for reasons other than pain.

TYPES OF SEDATIVE/HYPNOTIC DRUGS

The two major classes of sedatives/hypnotics are barbiturates and benzodiaz-epines. If any of the following drugs are prescribed to you to treat your chronic pain, you should ask your doctor for an alternative option.

Barbiturates

- Amobarbital (Amytal)
- Pentobarbital (Nembutal)
- Secobarbital (Seconal)
- Phenobarbitol (Luminal)

Benzodiazepines

- Alprazolam (Xanax)
- Chlordiazepoxide (Librium)
- Clonazepam (Klonopin)
- Diazepam (Valium)
- Estazolam (Prosom)
- Flunitrazepam (Rohypnol)
- Lorazepam (Ativan)
- Midazolam (Versed)
- Nitrazepam (Mogadon)
- Oxazepam (Serax)
- Temazepam (Restoril, Normison, Planum, Tenox, Temaze)
- Triazolam (Halcion)

Sedative Alert!

Chronic Side Effects of Sedatives/Hypnotics

- Prolonged cognitive impairment
- Chronic fatigue
- Onset or worsening of depression
- Tolerance (needing increasingly larger doses to maintain the same effect)
- Physical dependence (if taken regularly, the patient will need to slowly taper off the medicine to avoid withdrawal syndrome)

Sedative/hypnotic medication does not produce pain relief in patients with chronic pain and may cause both acute and chron-ic side effects. **Sedative/hypnotic drugs are bad medications for management of chronic pain and should not be prescribed.**

171

Alert! "Muscle Relaxants" Are Really Sedatives/Hypnotics

Note that we have put quotes around the term "muscle relaxants" because the drugs do not act directly on the muscle, but rather on the brain, much like the sedative/hypnotic drugs. They relax muscles by causing you to relax and feel tired. In fact, "muscle relaxants" are truly sedative/ hypnotic drugs. Like those drugs, "muscle relaxant" medications do not produce pain relief in chronic pain states, and often cause both acute and chronic side effects. **"Muscle relaxants" are generally bad medications for chronic pain.**

MUSCLE RELAXANTS ARE OKAY FOR ACUTE PAIN

Muscle relaxants are sometimes used to treat acute pain conditions, such as muscle problems associated with acute back pain. However, for a number of reasons, including their relatively poor pain-relieving capabilities and their potential side effects, these drugs are not typically recommended for chronic pain.

TYPES OF MUSCLE RELAXANTS (BRAND NAME)

- Carisprodol (Soma)
- Baclofen (Lioresal)
- Cyclobenzaprine (Flexeril)
- Dantrolene (Dantrium)
- Metaxalone (Skelaxin)
- Methocarbamol (Robaxin)
- Orphenadrine (Norflex)

Opioids' ("Narcotics") Historic Role

Opioid drugs are some of the oldest painkillers known to man. They have been used for thousands of years to treat all types of pain. Throughout time, and still today, no pain medication has had more controversy surrounding it than opioid drugs. It seems as though every decade there is a dramatic shift in medical wisdom as to what role these medications should play in the treatment of pain, especially chronic pain. In our medical careers, we have seen them play the role of both villain and superhero. In reality, they are more often the superhero than the villain, if prescribed appropriately to the right patient.

Besides being the drugs of choice for the treatment of acute moderate to severe pain from surgery or injury and for most types of cancer pain, opioid medication may also significantly relieve many patients' chronic pain. Over the past decade, lots of good scientific studies have shown that long-acting opioids can reduce the pain in some patients with low back pain, neuropathic pain, and arthritis pain.

Therefore, based on these studies and the experience of pain experts (like us), the vast majority of pain doctors feel that some patients with chronic pain can obtain significant pain relief from opioid medication, as long as they are prescribed and monitored properly (see "Who Is Appropriate for Opioid Medication?").

NAMES OF OPIOID DRUGS

Opioids can be divided into two groups, based on how long their action lasts in the body: short-acting opioids and long-acting opioids.

Short-Acting Opioid Drugs

- Tramadol (Ultram)
- Tramadol + acetaminophen (Ultracet)
- Codeine
- Oxycodone
- Oxycodone + acetaminophen (Percocet)
- Oxycodone + aspirin (Percodan)
- Hydrocodone + acetaminophen (Vicodin, Lortab)
- Morphine
- Meperedine (Demerol)
- Hydromorphone (Dilaudid)
- Oxymorphone IR (Opana IR)
- Transmucosal Fentanyl (Actiq, Fentora, Onsolis)
- Levorphanol

Long-Acting Opioid Drugs

- Tramadol ER (Ultram ER, Ryzolt)
- Long-acting morphine (MS Contin, Morphine ER, Embeda Kadian, Avinza)
- Methadone
- Long-acting hydromorphone (Exalgo)
- Long-acting oxycodone (Oxycontin, Oxycodone ER)
- Oxymorphone ER (Opana ER)
- Transdermal fentanyl patch (Duragesic)
- Levorphanol

OPIOID MEDICATION SIDE EFFECTS

Acute side effects

- Gastrointestinal issues (nausea, vomiting)
- Constipation
- Itchiness
- Cognitive problems (memory, concentration)

Chronic side effects

Although all of the following have been associated with long-term opioid use, not every patient will experience these side effects, and some may lessen with time:

- Constipation
- Sedation
- Irritability
- Cognitive problems (memory and concentration problems)
- Hypogonadism (decreased libido, irregular menstrual cycle, impotence)
- Rebound headaches

173

Help Stop Opioid Abuse

With the increased use of opioid medication to treat pain comes a societal cost. Specifically, some people take these drugs not to treat pain, but for their euphoric qualities. (Note that most pain patients do not experience euphoria from these drugs, but only find relief from the pain.) Taking opioid medication for euphoria can be very dangerous, if not fatal. When people overdose on these drugs—which is especially easy if they bite, chew, inject, or snort the long-acting opioids, such as Oxycontin, Opana ER, or Morphine ER—they can get a huge dose of the drug, causing them to stop breathing.

Studies have shown that the most common way nonpain persons get opioid pain medication is from a friend's or relative's medicine cabinet. Thus, one important way to stop the flow of opioid medication into society is to have a lock on your opioid medication and to dump it once you no longer need it. For the sake of the environment, please don't flush the pills down the toilet, but rather mix them with coffee grounds or cat litter and dispose of them in the garbage.

(continued)

WHO IS APPROPRIATE FOR OPIOID MEDICATION?

It is currently recommended that every chronic pain patient suffering from moderate to severe pain be viewed as a potential candidate for opioid therapy. The only issue concerns when the patient should be prescribed an opioid. Like most pain treatment experts today, we believe chronic opioid therapy should not be a first-line treatment and should be tried only after other nonopioid medications have been tried and have failed.

As opposed to old medical myths, some chronic pain patients with back pain, neuropathic pain, and OA pain find that opioid drugs actually provide the best balance of pain relief and side effects. In fact, opioids in some ways are safer for elderly patients than many other pain drugs, such as TCAs and antiseizure drugs.

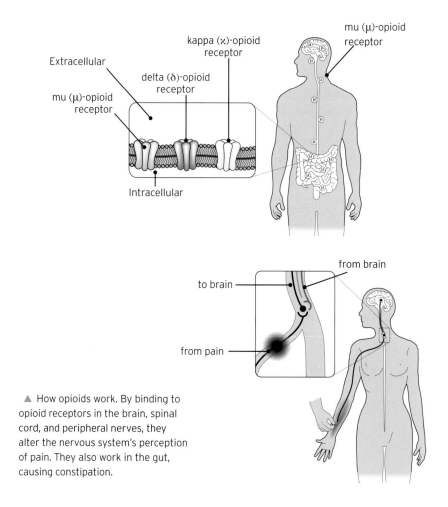

▲ How opioids work. By binding to opioid receptors in the brain, spinal cord, and peripheral nerves, they alter the nervous system's perception of pain. They also work in the gut, causing constipation.

Frequently Asked Questions About Opioids

HOW DO OPIOIDS WORK?

All animals, humans included, have natural chemicals (neurotransmitters) called *endorphins* and *enkaphalins* in our brain and spinal cord, where they play a vital role in reducing pain. More recently, these natural chemicals have also been found in our peripheral nerves and joints, where it is thought that they also work to reduce pain.

Opioid medications act just like our natural opioid-like neurotransmitters. They work in the same places as do our body's natural opiate chemicals, the endorphins and enkaphalins, within our spinal cord, brain, peripheral nerves, and joints, to help alleviate pain.

WHERE DO OPIOID DRUGS COME FROM?

There are several different types of opioid drugs:

- Natural opiates come from opium poppy resin and include morphine and codeine.
- Semisynthetic opioids are made using natural opiates and include hydromorphone, hydrocodone, oxycodone, and oxymorphone.
- Fully synthetic (man-made) opioids include fentanyl, methadone, and tramadol.
- Endogenous opioid chemicals are produced naturally in the body and include endorphins, enkephalins, dynorphins, and endomorphins.

DO OPIOIDS CAUSE ADDICTION IN CHRONIC PAIN PATIENTS?

First, we need to define what addiction is and is not. So many people confuse addiction with another biologic process, physical dependence. We're sure you have read the newspapers and seen on TV the accounts of people claiming to have become addicted to Oxycontin. Absolutely this is a major societal issue that needs to be dealt with. However, in our opinion, many of these folks on TV appeared not to be addicted, but rather had developed a physical dependence, which is a normal bodily reaction that happens with lots of different types of medication, including medications not used for pain, and is easily remedied.

(Help Stop Opioid Abuse continued)

FDA Steps In Because of all the issues with the abuse of opioid medication, the FDA has very appropriately instituted measures drug companies need to take while they are marketing these medications. The FDA has now required makers of opioid medications to institute risk-evaluation and mitigation strategies (REMS) to address the issues of abuse and misuse of these medications. Also, at the time of this writing, the FDA is contemplating a required learning course for all doctors who prescribe opioid medications and patients who take them, which we believe is a good idea.

What's New: Opioids that May Deter Abuse

Due to the societal issue of misuse of opioid drugs, drug companies have developed special formulations of their extended-release opioids that may make misuse less likely, and if abused, may less likely result in death.

How do these work? One drug recently approved by the FDA, Embeda, combines extended-release morphine with the anti-opioid naltrexone. Embeda results in the same amount of pain relief as morphine, but if the capsule is tampered with, naltrexone is released and works against the morphine, preventing death from respiratory depression.

Multiple other abuse-deterrent opioids are being developed with various other technologies, including pills that cannot be crushed.

Physical dependence is a natural occurrence that happens to everyone who takes certain drugs for a long period of time. Your body gets used to having the drug, so when you stop taking it, you will develop a negative withdrawal reaction. This happens not just with opioids, but also with nicotine, caffeine, alcohol, sedatives/hypnotics (e.g., Valium), antidepressants, blood pressure drugs, and steroids. Going into withdrawal after suddenly stopping an opioid does not mean you are addicted. Opioids, even if taken chronically, can be safely and comfortably stopped by gradually reducing the dosage, usually by 10 percent every five to seven days.

By definition, addiction is a psychological craving for a drug, and is apparent when a person takes an opioid for reasons other than pain relief. The addict lives every minute of the day thinking about how he or she will get his or her next dose of that drug. When chronic pain patients take opioids to treat their pain, they rarely develop a true addiction and drug craving. However, a risk factor for developing a true addiction to opioid medications, even if you are taking them for pain, is a history of a prior addiction, such as to alcohol or other drugs.

Pseudoaddiction Because of a Low Dose

Sometimes chronic pain patients may develop something called *pseudoaddiction*, which is caused by their doctor not appropriately prescribing the opioid medication. Pseudoaddiction happens when a patient's opioid medication is not being prescribed in doses strong enough to provide good pain relief, or the drug is not being prescribed often enough throughout the day. If this is the case, because the pain patient is still experiencing pain, he or she begins to take more doses than were prescribed to achieve good pain relief (and not for the high). Although this is a serious no-no, it is not a true addiction because the patient is not taking extra doses of the opioid medication to maintain a high, but rather is taking the extra pills to relieve pain. When a pseudoaddicted patient is prescribed the proper amount of opioid medication, he or she doesn't take any extra pills, because his or her pain is relieved.

Tolerance Is a Natural Reaction

Some pain patients (and even some of their doctors) mistakenly feel they are addicted because over time they need to take increasingly larger doses of the same opioid medication to experience the same amount of pain relief. This is called *tolerance*. Tolerance is a natural physical reaction and is not addiction. To be tolerant to opioids, a patient must first have demonstrated significant pain relief at a certain dose which remains stable for at least a month.

Also, in our experience, the issue of tolerance is overblown. Only a minority of chronic pain patients who are taking long-term opioids develop tolerance.

Physical Dependence

Physical dependence is not addiction! Lots of other non-narcotic drugs also produce a physical dependence, such as steroids, blood pressure medicine, and antidepressants. Physical dependence is another naturally occurring physical reaction that happens in everyone! All patients can safely be taken off opioid medication if the dose is slowly tapered down by their doctor.

The bottom line: Only rarely does opioid medication cause a true addiction when prescribed appropriately to a chronic pain patient who does not have a prior history of addiction.

HOW SHOULD OPIOID MEDICATION BE PRESCRIBED?

When using an opioid as one of the main treatments for chronic pain, long-acting opioid formulations are better than short-acting ones. Long-acting opioid medications should be prescribed around the clock, meaning that you take them at certain times on the clock (usually twice per day or once per day) and not based on how much pain you are feeling. This around-the-clock dosing results in a steady, constant amount of the drug in your blood, and therefore keeps you consistently more comfortable throughout the full twenty-four-hour cycle.

CONCLUSION: FIND THE DRUG THAT WORKS FOR YOU

As you have seen, you have an almost overwhelming number of medication options to consider when working with a doctor to treat your chronic pain. The appropriate choice will depend on your specific condition, the severity of the drug's side effects, and simply, what works best for you. In finding the ideal drug or drugs, it is important to remember to be patient and persistent. If the first one does not succeed, try and try again. It is critical for you to find a doctor who is familiar with how to prescribe all of these medications, and one who, like you, won't give up trying!

Q & A *with*
Dr. Argoff and Dr. Galer

I have nerve pain in my feet from diabetes. The doctor says there's not much to try except Percocet or Vicodin. Is this true?

No. While opioid narcotic medication, such as the oxycodone in Percocet and the hydrocodone in Vicodin, can alleviate all types of nerve pains, they are not the only medications that can treat neuropathic (nerve) pain and also likely shouldn't be the first medication to try most of the time. Nerve pains, whether from diabetes, shingles, or other types of nerve injury, can be successfully treated with many different types of drugs. While the FDA has approved only several medications to treat pain from diabetic neuropathy, including Pregabalin (Lyrica) and Duolexetine (Cymbalta), other drugs have been approved by FDA to treat Postherpetic Neuralgia, such as Lidocaine Patch (Lidoderm) and Gabapentin (Neurontin). Most pain experts agree that if a drug has been shown to treat one type of nerve pain problem it most likely can also help alleviate other kinds of nerve injury pains.

My doctor has kept me on the same medications to treat my pain for three years. I am not sure if they're helping me anymore. What should I do?

First, remember all medication changes must be reviewed with your doctor and she or he has to agree to such changes and monitor every change.

This is a very good question that many patients have or should be asking themselves. Any medications you take (whether for pain or any other condition) should only be taken if it is helping and not hurting you. For pain, that usually means that it is providing at least 30% pain relief and has no bad side effects. However, sometimes patients after a while aren't sure if the medication is working. The best way to tell is to see what happens as you slowly decrease the dose—does the pain get worse? Again, this must be done under your doctor's supervision. The good news is that if your current treatment is not helping you as much as in the past, it is likely that your doctor can consider a newer regimen that may be more helpful.

I am a 35-year-old with chronic back pain. Nothing has seemed to work, even two surgeries, nerve blocks, physical therapy, accupuncture and an electrical stimulator. I take Vicodin every once in a while and it really helps without any bad side effects. My doctor wants to put me on a strong opioid narcotic that I take every day, twice per day. I am afraid I'll become addicted, but the pain is just getting intolerable. What should I do?

Here are the facts. It is very uncommon for a person with chronic pain to become "addicted" to narcotics IF (1) he doesn't have a prior history of any addiction and (2) he only takes the medication to treat pain. Studies have shown that many chronic pain patients can experience significant pain relief with tolerable side effects from opioid narcotic medication when taken daily and no addiction. We definitely would try this type of treatment for our patients in your situation.

CHAPTER 9

Nerve Blocks and Other Interventions

Find the right treatment from the

variety of options.

Interventional approaches to pain reduction are often an important component of a comprehensive pain treatment program.

Like medications and other treatments, they often work best when used as part of a multimodal approach to treatment. By interventional approaches, we mean a medical procedure that is performed often through penetration of the skin.

- ✓ Trigger-point injections (TPIs)
- ✓ Nerve blocks
- ✓ Intravenous infusions and blocks
- ✓ Botulinum toxin injections
- ✓ Neurolytic blockades
- ✓ Nerve, spinal, and deep-brain stimulation
- ✓ Intraspinal analgesics

Intervention Basics

Two of the biggest challenges facing both you and your doctor are determining whether interventional pain management approaches are appropriate for you, and then determining which is best for you. Some procedures, such as facet joint injections with a cortisone-like substance and/or an anesthetic such as lidocaine, are designed to be effective for a short period of time; others, such as radiofrequency lesioning of the facet joint, are designed to last for several months.

Often, a doctor will first do the injection to determine if the area injected is a significant source of a person's pain complaint before doing a more long-lasting procedure such as radiofrequency lesioning. The more experienced and knowledgeable your doctor is about pain management, the more comfortable he or she will be in advising you regarding the appropriate procedure(s) for you.

Trigger-Point Injections Relieve Muscular Pain

Management of myofascial pain syndrome, the most common source of chronic back and neck pain, depends on elimination of painful myofascial trigger points. A variety of noninterventional treatments can be used to help accomplish this to the fullest extent possible, but often the early use of TPIs can help to improve your response to physical therapy (PT) and other nonmedicine approaches. TPIs are an interventional treatment to consider for this condition. For an experienced health care provider, these are easy and relatively safe to perform.

TPIS DISSOLVE THE TENSE KNOT

TPIs involve the placement of a needle into the trigger point and sometimes injecting a local anesthetic, a corticosteroid, or saline (salt water). Believe it or not, any of these or a combination of them (most often a local anesthetic combined with a steroid) can relax the trigger point at least temporarily and result in pain reduction. Some physicians who perform this injection have supported the use of dry-needling techniques in which nothing is injected, and an acupuncture needle is moved around to deactivate or break up the trigger point. This really does work! However, although success with dry-needling has been reported, we can tell you that patients are initially more comfortable when local anesthetics are used during the injection. Various local anesthetics can be used, including 0.5% procaine, 1% Lidocaine, or 0.25% bupivicaine. Some injections may be performed with a combination of these medications. Some injectors claim that certain herbal remedies such as an extract derived from the pitcher plant, sarapin, should be injected, although the mechanism of this herbal remedy is not known.

Intervention Alert!

Find an Experienced Doctor
Specific training is required for a doctor to perform each of these types of procedures, not only with respect to the procedure itself, but also with respect to the management of potential complications. **Always be willing to find out if the person who is recommending that you undergo a particular pain management procedure is trained appropriately. Don't be afraid or unwilling to ask!**

It is unclear whether the substance injected during a TPI significantly alters the response, and as we noted earlier, just putting a needle into the trigger point can deactivate it.

RELIEF FROM TPI LASTS FOR DAYS

We think that most often, the painful myofascial trigger point itself results from a chronic, perpetual, hyperexcitable state of both the peripheral and the central nervous systems, resulting in this painful neuromuscular syndrome. Myofascial TPIs can potentially interrupt this cycle of ongoing pain for an adequate time (usually days) to produce significant relief and improvement in function.

Typically, more than one trigger point is injected during each treatment session. The length of time injections provide relief is often measured in days; therefore, injections need to be offered as part of a comprehensive treatment program that includes therapeutic exercise, pharmacotherapy, and perhaps behavioral pain management approaches, as these therapies may be helpful in reducing myofascial pain. When TPIs provide relief that is so temporary so as not to be truly effective, we consider the use of botulinum toxin injections into the trigger points to prolong the benefit. This is an off-label use of this drug. The injection of botulinum toxin for any medical condition requires that the injector be well trained and experienced, so make sure of that before letting someone perform this procedure on you.

Nerve Blocks Interrupt the Pain Signal

Nerve blocks are procedures that are designed to interfere with normal nerve electrical activity to prevent or decrease pain. Remember that the nerves carry electrical information to the brain that may ultimately result in the experience of pain. Thus, a nerve block that interferes with this electrical activity may be able to reduce or eliminate the pain. The technique involves injecting a local anesthetic such as lidocaine or medications such as steroids, for example, cortisone and triamcinolone. Local anesthetics work primarily by blocking electrical activity within the nerve so that it can't send a pain signal to the brain. Steroids reduce inflammation and may also work in other ways to reduce pain.

How long do the pain-relieving effects of nerve blocks typically last? It is difficult to answer this question, as there is no typical response. Chronic pain management, even with nerve blocks, is not equivalent to chronic pain curing. Thus, nerve blocks will most likely provide a reduction of pain for days, weeks, and sometimes months, allowing you to use other pain-reducing activities (e.g., physical therapy and exercise) as well as to function more normally in general. Sometimes we perform nerve blocks to predict whether another more definitive procedure, such as radiofrequency lesioning, will work to provide longer-term relief.

NERVE BLOCKS CAN DIAGNOSE AND PREDICT PAIN

In addition to reducing pain, nerve blocks are often performed to help diagnose a painful condition, to predict what type of additional procedures may be best for you, and to prevent pain from occurring (e.g., after surgery). Four types of nerve blocks exist:

- **Diagnostic nerve blocks** may help your doctor to define the cause of pain and to better understand what type of pain may be present.
- **Prognostic nerve blocks** are performed to help predict the response to a different procedure that is being considered that may have a longer-lasting effect than a nerve block with a local anesthetic. For example, the face nerve pain condition known as *trigeminal neuralgia* is sometimes treated with interventional pain management approaches. A temporary trigeminal nerve block may be performed with a local anesthetic to help predict the patient's response to injection of a drug such as glycerol. Although glycerol injections may last a year or more, glycerol may produce side effects such as loss of sensation, since glycerol purposefully destroys parts of a nerve, and thus is known as a *neurolytic* or nerve-destroying agent.
- **Prophylactic nerve blocks**, also known as *preemptive analgesia*, are techniques performed to prevent pain from developing after surgery or trauma. This is a very exciting area of interventional pain management, since whenever possible we want to prevent acute pain from developing into chronic pain. Many pain specialists are working hard on treatments that one day may be able to routinely accomplish this. Considering that everyday acute pain syndromes associated with surgery or trauma are likely to occur and since acute pain may put a person at risk for developing chronic pain indefinitely, preventing this transformation of acute to chronic pain from occurring would be truly desirable.
- **Therapeutic nerve blocks** may be used in either acute or chronic pain syndrome to reduce pain and help a person get back to full activity when combined with a therapeutic exercise program. For example, if you were experiencing severe low back and leg pain as the result of a herniated disc compressing a nerve root in your lower back, an epidural injection of steroid medication could relieve enough pain for you to participate in a PT program so that you could help strengthen your back and maintain your activity at as normal a level as possible.

Get the Facts: Chronic Pain Syndromes That Can Possibly Benefit from Nerve Blocks

- Myofascial pain syndromes
- Painful scars
- Neuromas (a collection of nerve endings that develops after surgery or trauma)
- Degenerative joint syndromes such as osteoarthritis and sacroiliac joint dysfunction
- Spinal degenerative conditions such as facet syndromes, degenerative or herniated discs, and nerve root compression
- Chronic headaches

Note: Nerve blocks for chronic pain generally do not "cure" the problem, but when combined with other treatments they may result in a more manageable pain level and improved function. If you are advised to have a nerve block, expect that the benefits will not last forever.

183

Adverse Side Effects of Nerve Blocks

- Allergic reactions to the medication(s) used that, if severe, can result in death (but most commonly they're not that severe)
- Toxic or excessive blood levels of the local anesthetic or other medications used, resulting in side effects including dizziness, sedation, and heart rhythm abnormalities
- Unintended injury to nerve or non-nerve structures that can result in problems such as paralysis, loss of sensation, and tendon injury
- Increased pain and anxiety-related reactions

Serious side effects are uncommon. Usually, a patient will experience increased pain for a day or two at the site of the nerve block before he or she truly experiences the benefits of the injection.

Nerve Blocks for Various Pains

PARAVERTEBRAL NERVE BLOCKS LOCATE THE PAIN

Paravertebral nerve blocks are used diagnostically to determine the precise nerve roots or segments responsible for the pain caused by a herniated disks; osteophytes, another spinal degenerative conditions; a tumors; or a vascular lesion. They are performed in the cervical, thoracic, lumbar, or sacral region. They can help predict whether patients who are being considered for neurostimulation or a neurolytic procedure (we describe both of these below) are good candidates for these procedures, and also therapeutically to provide temporary relief of pain in the affected region.

Regardless of where the paravertebral block is performed, there is a risk of the injection going into areas around the spine such as the epidural or subarachnoid spaces, which can result in certain neurological functions being diminished. These may range from temporary loss of sensation or loss of strength to the inability to breathe on one's own. In the thoracic region, pneumothorax (air inside the thoracic cavity that has led to a complete or partial collapsed lung) is one of the more common complications.

OCCIPITAL NERVE BLOCKS FIGHT HEADACHES

Occipital nerve blocks can lessen the pain associated with a variety of chronic headache syndromes, including migraines, occipital neuralgia (a nerve pain condition located in the back of the head), and cervicogenic headaches (headaches caused by cervical spine disorders). This injection is performed most often as an office procedure and involves the injection of a local anesthetic with or without a steroid (depending on the training of the person doing the injection).

The occipital nerve runs on the left and right sides of the back of your head, just lateral to the middle of the back of your head. There are few complications, and the immediate results can be gratifying for the person receiving the injection—as well as the person doing the injection because the patient may report dramatic pain relief right away! This procedure can easily be performed in the office. Although it often provides temporary relief, in our experience this injection does not provide long-term benefits.

INTERCOSTAL NERVE BLOCKS FOR THE CHEST AND ABDOMEN

Intercostal nerve blocks may be used for diagnostic or therapeutic reasons. They help to define and manage pain associated with chest and abdominal wall processes such as intercostal neuralgia (pain due to irritability of the nerves located around the ribs) and other syndromes. They are particularly helpful for the relief of acute post-traumatic or postsurgical pain in the thoracic or abdominal wall.

For chronic pain, intercostal nerve blocks may be used to treat the pain following shingles: postherpetic neuralgia (PHN), or the condition known as intercostal neuralgia. Some pain specialists will consider destroying the affected intercostal nerves by cryoanalgesia (freezing the nerve) or radiofrequency lesioning (heating the nerve to destroy its ability to carry pain information). Although excellent temporary relief is obtained after a local anesthetic intercostal block, to provide a greater duration of benefit cryoanlagesia or radiofrequency lesioning may be recommended when the local anesthetic nerve block stops working.

SYMPATHETIC NERVE BLOCKS CAN HELP SOME WITH REFLEX SYMPATHETIC DYSTROPHY/COMPLEX REGIONAL PAIN SYNDROME (RSD/CRPS)

Sympathetic nerve blocks are an important treatment modality for some patients with CRPS Type 1 or II (RSD or causalgia, respectively). Both conditions are associated with hyperalgesia (more pain than usually experienced when a normally painful sensation is applied, such as pinching), allodynia (pain following a normally nonpainful sensation, such as covering the feet with a sheet), burning pain, and varying degrees of vascular (cool, bluish extremities) and sweating abnormalities (see chapter 4).

For some patients with RSD/CRPS, sympathetic nerve blocks can be an effective therapeutic modality, especially if they are performed soon after onset and are combined with other noninterventional treatments such as PT. The sympathetic nerves have different control towers, or ganglia, in different parts of the body. The duration of benefit from sympathetic nerve blocks is variable depending on a number of factors, including how soon after the onset of pain the injections are performed (the sooner the better) and whether the pain is completely controlled by the sympathetic nerves.

Temporarily Block Your Shoulder Pain

The suprascapular nerve provides sensation to the supraspinatus muscle around your shoulder blade and shoulder joint. Therefore, a suprascapular nerve block can temporarily relieve shoulder joint pain and allow a person with certain severe shoulder pain syndromes to perform active range-of-motion exercises. Frozen shoulder syndrome as a result of immobilization (e.g., following a motor vehicle accident or a stroke) may be prevented by this procedure.

185

We have learned over many years that people with pain caused by the sympathetic nervous system may also be experiencing nerve injury–related or neuropathic pain due to other types of nerves. This adds dramatically to the complexity of treating people with this kind of pain problem and likely explains why sympathetic blocks do not work for all people. There is still no "cure" at this time for all RSD/CRPS-related pain, but much can be done to relieve a noticeable amount of it.

Cervicothoracic (stellate ganglion), celiac plexus, splanchnic (gut), and lumbar sympathetic blocks are the names of some of the anatomic regions where sympathetic blocks can be performed. Other conditions that have been treated with sympathetic nerve blocks include postamputation pain, peripheral vascular disease, pain associated with pancreatitis or pancreatic cancer, acute herpetic neuralgia (shingles), and PHN. Various other cancer pain syndromes have also been treated with this modality.

Measuring the effect of a sympathetic block may involve measuring changes in skin temperature or skin sweating, because the sympathetic nervous system as part of its normal function regulates skin temperature and sweating.

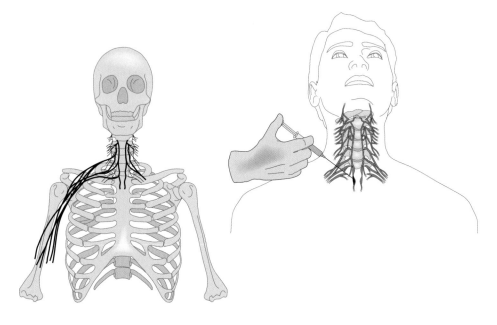

▲ Cervical Sympathetic Nerve Block
(also called Stellate Ganglion Nerve
Block and Brachial Plexus Nerve Block)

BRACHIAL PLEXUS NERVE BLOCKS REDUCE PAIN IN ARMS

The brachial plexus is a collection of nerves leaving your cervical spine that come together around your collarbone and travel down to your arms. The brachial plexus can be injured following trauma, as the result of cancer invasion, and in a number of other settings such as following an operation or after a vaccination. When injured, it can result in severe pain. Brachial plexus blocks can be useful in controlling such pain as well as pain due to CRPS; shoulder–hand syndrome after stroke; acute herpetic neuralgia (shingles); PHN involving areas supplied by the C5–T1 nerve roots; pain associated with the vascular insufficiency of Raynaud's disease; and phantom limb pain. Brachial plexus blocks may allow for greater range-of-movement exercises for people with a frozen shoulder, elbow, or wrist. They also may be used for postoperative pain management and the prevention of phantom limb pain after amputation.

Intravenous Nerve Blocks

As the name implies, intravenous nerve blocks are performed through an intravenous route. One such block, named after the anesthesiologist who developed it, is called a *Bier block*. With the Bier block, the limb to be treated is isolated from the rest of the systemic circulation using a tourniquet, and then various medications may be injected into the limb intravenously for pain relief.

If CRPS is suspected, some specialists may want you to undergo an intravenous phentolamine infusion. This medication can block the sympathetic nervous system, so it may be helpful in determining if the sympathetic nervous system is causing the pain. In our experience, use of intravenous phentolamine is potentially effective, not only to help diagnose CRPS but also as a treatment for it.

Intravenous or subcutaneous (infused just under the skin) lidocaine, administered either as one several-hour treatment or on an ongoing basis, can be helpful for a wide variety of chronic pain syndromes, including CRPS, PHN, peripheral neuropathy pain, central neuropathic pain, myofascial pain, and fibromyalgia.

EPIDURAL STEROID INJECTIONS (ESI)

The epidural space is the outermost portion of the spinal canal, running essentially the entire length of the spine. ESIs involve the injection of a steroid into the epidural space at any level of the spine. Steroids have potent anti-inflammatory as well as pain-relieving properties.

Relieve Your Thigh Pain

Meralgia parasthetica is the medical term used to describe pain and abnormal, unpleasant sensations along the thigh in the distribution of the lateral femoral cutaneous nerve. This syndrome is commonly associated with obesity, weight loss (e.g., after pregnancy), diabetes, or tight belts. A lateral femoral cutaneous nerve block is sometimes useful for treatment of this syndrome.

187

Many pain specialists have suggested a series of three injections as a treatment; however, no good data exists to confirm that three are better than two or one. Some people may, in fact, do better with one or two, and others with three.

In any case, no more than six injections should be done within a twelve-month period. Although many pain specialists perform this procedure without radiologic guidance, reports of needle placement errors within the epidural space have demonstrated that for some patients, the use of fluoroscopic (X-ray) guidance and contrast material (injected into the epidural space during the procedure to determine that the needle is truly in the epidural space) may be wisest.

How Are ESIs Used?

Most often, ESIs are used to treat low back and leg pain associated with a condition known as *lumbosacral radiculopathy*. Patients are referred for these injections with diverse causes of their back pain, ranging from spinal stenosis to bulging disks to herniated disks to simple back sprain. Conditions involving the nerve leaving the spine are most likely to be effectively treated by ESIs.

These injections are not as helpful for patients who have low back pain only. Many areas of the spine, including nerve roots, spinal nerves, bony elements, and connective tissue, may be subjected to prolonged inflammatory states, stretching, or ischemia. Orthopedists and neurosurgeons often rely on ESIs to help reduce the spine-related pain of patients who they do not believe are clear surgical candidates. Short-term benefit (two to four weeks) from these injections is commonly observed, but long-term benefit is not seen as often.

Cervical epidural injections of steroids are indicated primarily for neck pain associated with cervical spine degenerative disc disease. Pain as a consequence of spinal stenosis, which leads to a narrowed intervertebral foramen, or a pre-existing osteoarthritic disorder, may be treated with cervical ESIs.

Enough Is Enough!

When you are using ESIs remember that more is not better. A steroid formulation such as methylprednisolone or triamcinolone is usually injected in doses of 40–80 mg every two to four weeks, with a maximum of three injections in six months. The best current evidence suggests that additional injections offer no clear additional benefit, and they may increase the risk of side effects.

Our adrenal gland is normally responsible for making most of our body's steroids, but when we are exposed to steroids through injections (through oral medications such as prednisone or through oral supplements) the adrenal gland sometimes becomes suppressed and stops making its own steroids. Adrenal suppression with decreased cortisol (steroid) levels has been shown to occur for three to five weeks after a typical ESI in some patients, although it is not common. If this does occur, the adrenal gland may need to be "coaxed' back into making steroids again. Also, multiple injections may produce injury to the spinal ligaments.

Complications of the procedure include epidural hematoma (bleeding in the epidural space), infection, and post-procedure headache. Adverse effects of the steroids include hypertension, congestive heart failure, abnormal menses, adrenal gland abnormalities, paralysis, ligament injury, osteoporosis, low cortisol levels, and fluid retention. Stroke and respiratory failure is an uncommon complication of cervical spine epidural injections.

FACET JOINT INJECTIONS FOR BACK AND NECK PAIN

The source of chronic low back and/or neck pain may be located in the facet joints; the facet joints are located between and behind adjacent vertebrae (back bones) and help stabilize the back during movement. Pain due to facet disease increases with extension, rotation, or lateral movement of the spine, and is most often deep in the paravertebral regions of the back or neck. The facet joint has a special sensory nerve supply that is fed by branches of spinal nerves above and below the affected joint. Overgrowth of bone in this region (osteophytes) and other degenerative changes in these joints are thought to contribute to the pain.

A local anesthetic block of the medial branch nerve within the facet joint helps to make the diagnosis of facet joint pain. The addition of a steroid to these injections may provide prolonged relief. Cryoanalgesia (freezing the area) or radiofrequency neurolysis (nerve destruction) of the medial branch nerve in the facet joint may be considered if the local anesthetic block gives adequate but only temporary pain relief.

Botulinum Toxin Injections

Botulinum toxin injections are used off label for a growing number of painful conditions including cervical dystonia, spasticity, chronic myofascial pain, chronic low back pain, whiplash-associated pain, temporomandibular joint dysfunction, neuropathic pain, and chronic headache. Serious side effects are uncommon and include pain and weakness at the injection site, bleeding, infection, and the development of flu-like symptoms within the first two days following treatment.

Botox Approved in the UK for Treatment of Migraines

As this book was going to press, the UK government approved the use of Botox for the treatment of migraine headaches.

In clinical studies, migraine patients were given up to five courses of Botox injections into specific head and neck muscles every 12 weeks.

After one year of treatment, almost 70 percent of those treated with Botox had a 50 percent reduction in the number of migraines. This use of Botox is not yet approved by the FDA.

189

What's New: Intradiscal Electrothermal (IDET) Annuloplasty Warms the Disc

IDET is a minimally invasive procedure currently being used most commonly for management of chronic low back pain caused by lumbar degenerative disc disease.

How is it done? This procedure requires significant technical expertise, as a wire needs to be placed under the skin and then around a disc so that heat can be used to treat the injured disc.

What are the results? This is a new procedure that is still not widely used. Some recent studies question the long-term efficacy with this intervention.

Are there any side effects? Immediate side effects are rare; long-term side effects are unknown.

Botulinum toxins are potent agents that prevent various nerve chemicals, called *neurotransmitters*, from being released at nerve endings. Recently it's been found that botulinum toxins have an effect on multiple chemicals and neurotransmitters in the nervous system that are involved in the perception of pain, including acetylcholine, glutamate, calcitonin gene-related peptide, and Substance P.

The recent discovery that botulinum toxin not only stops muscles from contracting but also can relieve pain led researchers to look for why this may be the case. Although it was known for many years that botulinum toxin affected the chemical acetylcholine, which resulted in reduced muscle contraction, the discovery that botulinum toxin affects three other nerve chemicals is startling; these nerve chemicals are important for pain transmission to occur, and therefore their inhibition by botulinum toxin may help to explain why pain relief occurs.

There are several strains of botulinum toxin types: A–F. Three types of botulinum toxin are currently available in the United States: two type A toxins (Botox and Dysport) and one type B toxin (Myobloc). Without a doubt, Botox has been the most extensively studied botulinum toxin in the United States, especially with respect to its effect on pain reduction.

Neurolytic Blockades Using Chemicals, Cold, and Heat

Neurolytic blockade is the term used to describe the process by which neurons (nerves) are purposefully damaged to produce a desired clinical effect. Neurolytic blockade can be accomplished through injected chemicals (phenol, glycerol, or alcohol), the use of cold (cryotherapy), or the use of heat (radiofrequency lesioning). Because of the damage done by neurolytic blocks, these should most often only be performed on patients with cancer pain and a limited amount of life expectancy, with a few exceptions such as for trigeminal neuralgia.

CHEMICAL BLOCKS ARE UNPREDICTABLE

The use of chemical agents often produces nonselective, significant nerve damage that cannot be controlled; therefore, the risk of increased pain due to the nerve injury that may be produced is clear. Neurolytic blocks with chemical agents are most often reserved for use in intractable pain states or in terminal illnesses such as cancer-related pain.

CRYOANALGESIA PUTS PAIN ON ICE

Cooling a nerve is known to produce a reversible nerve block; nerve fibers that control touch and those that control pain are particularly susceptible to cold-induced damage. The term *cryoanalgesia* refers to the destruction of peripheral nerves by cold, and this procedure is performed to achieve pain control. It has been used for intractable cancer pain, facial pain, post-thoracotomy pain, and other types of chest pain. The duration of pain relief following cryoanalgesia may range from as little as two days to seven months or longer.

RADIOFREQUENCY LESIONING BURNS AWAY THE PAIN

Radiofrequency ablation (sometimes termed *lesioning*) is a procedure that uses a thermal (temperature) probe and a radiofrequency generator (a machine to generate heat) to selectively injure certain nerve fibers for pain control.

Currently, radiofrequency ablation is commonly used for various spinal pain disorders, including pain of facet or discogenic origin in the facet joints and spinal discs, as well as for sympathetically maintained pain and trigeminal neuralgia.

Although nerves are destroyed during this procedure, the destructive effect is less than when chemicals such as phenol or glycerol are used to destroy nerves, and as a result, the risk of increased pain following the procedure is less than when chemicals are used for neurolysis.

Electrical Stimulation Of The Nerves, Spine, And Brain

PERIPHERAL NERVE STIMULATION (PNS) BLOCKS SENSORY NERVES

In the peripheral nervous system (arms, legs, and trunk), electrical stimulation has been shown to block certain types of sensory nerves. Central nervous system effects of PNS have also been reported. Studies have reported benefit of PNS in neuropathic pain including CRPS, and postsurgical low back and radicular (nerve root) pain.

The peripheral nerve stimulator is first used on a trial basis to determine its effectiveness. The trial period can last a varying amount of time, from days to a week or so. If the PNS is helpful enough and there are no adverse effects, the system may be implanted or placed under the skin so that nothing is visible on top of the skin. The patient can turn the stimulator on and off through a special magnet. This is a highly specialized treatment, so make sure the practitioner offering this to you has experience with it! Adverse effects include bleeding, infection, wire migration (if the wires move out of position, they will not provide the same benefit), and battery failure.

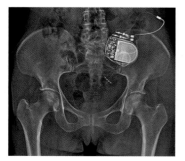

▲ Spinal Stimulator

SPINAL CORD STIMULATION REPLACES PAIN WITH TINGLING

Spinal stimulation techniques require the placement of electrical leads in the epidural space that are designed to stimulate the spinal cord so that an area of pain is "covered" or replaced by a nonpainful tingling or other sensation. The exact mechanism of action of spinal cord stimulation is not known, but it is believed that it involves the activation of pain-modulating mechanisms that dampen pain transmission.

Pain due to nerve injury (neuropathic pain), including spinal as well as non-spinal etiologies, remains the most common reason for using spinal stimulation. It has also been used in chronic low back pain without radiation to the lower extremities, as well as neck and thoracic spine pain. It can also control the painful sensations that can be experienced by individuals with multiple sclerosis.

As with PNS, a trial period is required for spinal cord stimulators. If you are a potential candidate for spinal cord stimulation, you must be able to understand how to regulate the stimulation, as successful treatment will depend on your ability to adjust and regulate the stimulator. You will be taught how to do this during the trial period.

This treatment is more often partially effective as opposed to being completely effective in relieving pain. Currently, there is great interest in the potential benefit of this modality for the management of pain due to peripheral vascular disease (lack of blood flow to the lower extremities) and for the management of chest pain due to coronary artery disease.

DEEP BRAIN STIMULATION MAY RELIEVE NEUROPATHIC PAIN

Deep brain stimulation refers to the direct electrical stimulation of various targets in the brain to reduce pain. Very sophisticated surgical techniques are used to place the electrodes in the desired areas of the brain. No large studies exist to document its role in pain control; however, stimulation of brain areas responsible for motor activity appears to be a possible treatment for patients suffering from severe central or trigeminal neuropathic pain who have not benefited from other, less-invasive techniques.

Intraspinal Analgesic Therapy Provides Constant Pain Relief

Intraspinal opiates have been used in the management of cancer-related pain for several decades; more recently, their use in the management of chronic, noncancer-related pain has been established as well. Intraspinal infusion systems are appropriate for patients with chronic pain who have not benefited from other systemic and/or interventional/noninterventional therapies.

Several types of implantable medication infusion systems exist, including those that provide a constant flow and dose as well as those that are programmable so that the infusion dose can be adjusted. Each type requires proper patient selection, a trial of intraspinal analgesia prior to implantation, and long-term follow-up. Catheter and pump failures, although not common, are not rare either.

Medications that have been used in such infusion systems include morphine; other opioids; ziconotide, a potent, nonopioid pain medication; and baclofen, which is especially helpful for spasticity reduction. The use of various combinations of agents, such as an opiate and a local anesthetic together, is common in clinical practice, although such combinations haven't been well studied for efficacy nor safety.

CONCLUSION

It's exciting that so many interventional pain management treatments are available to help relieve some patients with chronic pain. However, they need to be used for the right person by the right doctor and as part of a comprehensive approach to the management of pain. Before you have any procedure, as with a medicine, you need to make sure the doctor is appropriately trained and experienced, you are the right type of patient for the procedure, and you need to make sure you understand the possible risks and true benefits of the intervention recommended.

CHAPTER 10

Active Physical Therapy is Essential

Avoid "feel good" therapy that fails to reverse the underlying problem.

the PRESCRIPTION for PHYSICAL THERAPY (PT)

In our several decades' worth of treating chronic pain, we have repeatedly seen how important appropriate PT treatments can be to so many of our patients.

Honestly, in medical school and in our neurology training, we were not taught about the importance of PT. Therefore, it is likely that many of your doctors are also ignorant of its critical role in treating chronic pain. Hopefully, this chapter will arm you with information that you can take to your doctor to discuss how to obtain appropriate PT for your condition.

✓ Active PT (absolutely critical)
✓ Passive PT (feels good, but is less important)

Get the Facts: Parts of an Active PT Program

An active PT program should include the following components:
- Muscle/tendon/ligament stretching and strengthening
- Aerobic exercise
- Weight bearing on the painful body part
- Normal movements of the involved body region

The Most Common Reasons an Active PT Program Fails

- Your program is not designed or managed by a physical therapist trained to treat your specific condition.
- You fail to do your homework. (A good active PT program should include home-based daily activities: your "homework.")
- At home, you base your level of activity/exercise on how you're feeling:
  - On "good days" you do too much activity.
  - On "bad days" you don't do enough activity.

Active Versus Passive PT

Not only are most doctors untrained in the most appropriate types of PT for chronic pain, so are most physical therapists, believe it or not! Most therapists are trained in only "passive" PT modalities, in which the treatment is done to the patient: massage, ultrasound, hydrotherapy, etc. Although these treatments can definitely make you feel better while you are receiving them, they should not have a major role in most patients' treatment regimens. They will not have any meaningful effect in reversing or improving the underlying problem. Passive treatments may be used sparingly and should play a minor role in relieving chronic pain. The only real downsides to passive PT are the costs and wasted time you could be spending on more important, active forms of PT.

"Active" PT modalities are crucial to a successful outcome for back pain, neck pain, arthritis, Reflex Sympathetic Dystrophy/Complex Regional Pain Syndrome (RSD/CRPS), and fibromyalgia. By definition, an "active" PT program is one in which the patient is trained in specific exercises to address his or her specific needs. It usually is not just a general exercise program, but rather is tailored to the patient's chronic pain condition and his or her abilities. Also, the program's pace—the progression of activity—should be gradual and slow.

It is critical to find a physical therapist who is trained and has experience treating your specific chronic pain condition.

Active PT Provides Long-Lasting Results

An active PT program is probably the most essential component of treatment for most patients with back pain, neck pain, osteoarthritis, RSD/CRPS, and fibromyalgia. Although some patients with lesser disabilities may do well in a "normal person" regular exercise program, such as in a gym or pool, most chronic pain patients need to be evaluated and treated by a physical therapist who is specifically trained and experienced in designing and executing a specific active PT program for their condition. You must ask if your therapist has this training, as most do not!

A QUOTA TO MEASURE IMPROVEMENT

A graded, quota-based progression system is critical to the success of an active PT program. For each activity or exercise, a baseline is obtained to determine what the patient can do comfortably without increased pain or fatigue. The patient then begins the program doing only 75 percent of this baseline level for each activity or exercise. Then, over the course of the program, the patient increases the number and/or length of time of each activity or exercise by 5 percent to 10 percent every five days to two weeks, depending on the patient. The key, regardless of your age or condition, is to stick to the plan, regardless of pain level.

Passive PT Relieves Pain Briefly

MASSAGE RELAXES MUSCLES

We all know how great a massage can feel. And with chronic myofascial pain conditions, such as back and neck pain, a massage done by an experienced therapeutic massage therapist can make you feel better almost immediately. However, your tight and spastic muscles will return to their abnormal state if you do not also pair your massages with an active PT program.

ULTRASOUND HEATS UP THE MUSCLES

Ultrasound in our minds is a very questionable technique for the treatment of chronic pain. It reportedly works by creating high-frequency sound waves to create heat in muscles and tissues underneath the probe on the skin. Some people claim that the heat increases the blood flow into these tissues and makes them healthier. We don't recommend that this therapy be continued indefinitely for our patients with chronic pain because we don't see any long-term benefits. There are no side effects, but again, remember that you need to be time- and cost-sensitive. Make the best use of your time and money!

HYDROTHERAPY PUTS PAIN IN WATER

Hydrotherapy can mean lots of things. Most often, hydrotherapy means you or your pained body part is placed in a whirlpool-like bath, where the temperature of the water is adjusted for heating or cooling. This may feel wonderful, but in our opinion hydrotherapy provides minimal long-term benefit. (However, for some PT programs, hydrotherapy can mean exercise in a pool, which is a form of "active" PT, which we do recommend.)

PARAFFIN WAX TREATMENT DRIPS HEAT ON SKIN

Paraffin wax treatment was actually used by the Romans to treat injuries and pain. Typically, you put your pained body part into a warm bath of wax, like dipping a candle. Similar to ultrasound and warm hydrotherapy, this form of passive PT supposedly helps the patient by warming up the local tissues. Again, it feels great, but there's not much long-term benefit.

DESENSITIZATION RUBS AWAY PREVIOUS PAIN

Desensitization is very useful for chronic pain conditions that involve severe skin sensitivity (allodynia), such as RSD/CRPS. The actual process of desensitization may seem a bit barbaric, but it does work. The patient rubs the painful skin region with unpleasant objects, such as an object that would be benign for most of us, like a piece of cloth, a hairbrush, or Velcro, which helps the nervous system

Iontophoresis Is Obsolete

An iontophoresis device is a machine that uses electrical current on the skin to deliver medicines, such as steroids and nonsteroidal anti-inflammatory drugs, into the soft tissues. The electrical stimulation helps to open the pores in the skin and drive chemicals/drugs past the skin barrier and into the underlying tissues. However, we believe iontophoresis is a waste of time and money now that FDA-approved topical drugs are available, which allow the patient to do the same thing at home on a daily basis.

197

What's New: Using Mirrors Can Produce Dramatic Effects

Over the past several years, studies have been published demonstrating how mirror therapy can have dramatic positive effects for patients who are living with certain types of chronic pain. In particular, patients with RSD/CRPS of a limb and those with phantom limb pain can experience dramatic improvement in their pain by literally just looking into a mirror.

How does it work? Working with a trained physical therapist, the patient adjusts the mirror so that it appears that he or she is moving the painful limb, but in reality is moving the nonpainful limb. It's really a way to trick the brain into believing the painful limb is moving without pain. And it works! Although the reason this works is still unknown, several studies have shown that using this technique at least once per day for several weeks can produce dramatic results. And there are no side effects! We strongly suggest that folks with RSD/CRPS of a limb or phantom limb pain try it.

readapt to the skin being touched and stimulated. As the patient tolerates one object, a different object is used (objects can differ in texture, vibration, and temperature). With all of these different types of stimulation, the aim is to reset the nerves and brain into "feeling" these things once again. Just as when you are learning or relearning any skill or sport, you have to start with small skill sets, and gradually learn harder and more complex tasks. This commonly used technique of gradually increasing the degree of complexity helps your nervous system (nerves, spinal cord, and brain) to become accustomed to any type of new stimuli.

TENS PUTS THE POWER IN THE PATIENT'S HAND

TENS is a portable machine in which low-energy electrical current is delivered through electrodes that are placed around the painful body part. One theory of how TENS works is that it stimulates certain types of peripheral nerves in the area to block the pain signal as it goes into the spinal cord. However, others think TENS may help some people with certain localized pain by producing a buzzing/tingling sensation that then distracts the patient from the pain. Regardless of how it works, we believe it may be useful to try on patients with back and neck pain, especially since there are no side effects. Usually, a two- to four-week trial is all that's needed to see if it works for a patient. As with medicines, this helps some patients and not others, and there is no way to predict who will benefit from it.

CONCLUSION: FIND THE RIGHT ACTIVE PHYSICAL THERAPIST

For many patients with chronic pain, participating in the correct PT program is as important, if not more important, than any medicine or procedure. The key to getting the right program for you is to find a physical therapist who is trained in treating your chronic pain condition. One place to look is at the closest medical center's multidisciplinary pain clinic.

CHAPTER 11

Psychological Treatments for Everyone

Specialized techniques help

people with chronic pain.

the PRESCRIPTION *for* MENTAL HEALTH

Even if you are one of the lucky ones who do not have a psychological condition as a result of your chronic pain, you still can benefit greatly from certain psychological techniques that are designed to help all people with chronic pain.

Although in certain cases psychotherapy may be important and helpful to some patients, we will not be emphasizing this "talk therapy." Rather, we are going to focus on techniques that can benefit the vast majority of chronic pain patients. These are well-proven, fairly simple ways a trained pain psychologist can help you retrain your brain with new ways of thinking about your pain that often have a huge positive impact on both your pain and your ability to function.

- ✓ Relaxation therapy
- ✓ Imagery
- ✓ Biofeedback
- ✓ Cognitive-behavioral therapy
- ✓ Hypnosis

Chronic Pain Often Leads to Depression and Anxiety

The unfortunate fact is that many people with chronic pain will at some time suffer from a psychological disorder due to their pain and disability. The psychological conditions they experience are usually depression or an anxiety disorder. Less often, some chronic pain patients will suffer from a particular type of anxiety disorder: post-traumatic stress disorder (PTSD), especially if their pain was caused by or is associated with a traumatic event.

It's important to recognize that these psychological conditions do not cause chronic pain and are not the reason you have pain, but rather reflect the devastating effects of living your life in chronic pain.

Seek Treatment for Major Depression

Depression is divided into two types: minor depression and major depression. Most people with chronic pain at some time in their life will experience a minor depression. However, a major depression is a serious medical condition that needs to be treated with medication, with the nonmedication treatments we outline in this chapter, or with both.

DEPRESSION IS COMMON AND NATURAL

It makes complete common sense that if you live most of every day with chronic pain you are at risk for developing depression. Just knowing the pain will be there every morning when you wake up and every night when you go to bed is enough to raise anyone's risk of developing depression (and anxiety). And then, if you add the "tsunami of pain" (see chapter 14)—such as the disability most people have with their pain, how pain can affect your relationships, how sometimes doctors, insurance companies, and workers' compensation systems don't believe you, and so forth—you can really understand why chronic pain patients are prone to developing depression. In fact, we think those who don't become at least somewhat depressed must be superhuman!

What makes matters worse is that the depression can actually make your pain feel worse, and your pain makes you more depressed. Also, both of these conditions can interfere with sleep, which in turn can worsen both pain and depression. This bad concoction of pain, depression, and poor sleep is very common in patients with chronic pain. If you are in this horrible vicious cycle, remember that you are not alone, though you may feel like you are. Because this bad blend of symptoms is so common, many well-known treatments are available that can

Signs of Major Depression

A major depression is diagnosed when a person has five or more of the following symptoms for at least two weeks:

- Feeling sad, hopeless, worthless, or pessimistic
- Behavior changes, such as new eating and sleeping patterns
- A loss of interest in things that were meaningful to the patient in the past

What's New: Depression and Pain Share Brain Chemistry

Every year, more and more studies are published in the medical literature showing how closely depression and pain are tied with regard to their underlying causes within the brain.

How are they connected?

For decades now, it's been known that depression and pain share similar brain chemicals: serotonin and norepinephrine. Thus, many drugs that are used to treat pain are also used to treat depression (and vice versa), such as the older tricyclic antidepressants (TCAs) and the newer duloxetine (Cymbalta). More recently, brain imaging studies using functional magnetic resonance imaging and positron emission tomography scans have shown that there is much overlap in the brain areas involved in the feeling of pain and the emotions associated with it, and the brain regions involved in depression.

make a significant positive impact when prescribed and performed by experienced pain health care providers. Each of the common psychological disorders needs treatment, but depression needs a full-court press.

Anxiety Disorders Cause Unreal Fear

Anxiety disorders are a group of conditions that cause irrational, unhealthy, persistent, and excessive anxiety, worry, and fear—unfounded, ungrounded fear. Some patients may have a chronic longstanding anxiety that existed prior to their pain, while others have so-called panic attacks, which are sudden attacks of severe anxiety and terror. Panic attacks cause the "fight or flight" stress reaction due to adrenaline overload: a pounding heart, sweating, weakness, faintness, and lightheadedness. During these attacks, people's limbs may tingle or feel numb, and some people may experience nausea, chest pain, or smothering sensations. Panic attacks also usually cause a sense of unreality, a feeling of impending doom, or a fear of losing control.

Though depression is often thought of as being the most common psychiatric disorder to co-occur with chronic pain, studies have shown that anxiety disorders occur at least as often. Like depression, anxiety can worsen pain and also interfere with sleep. Also, as with depression, an anxiety disorder must be treated as a significant problem, apart from the chronic pain.

PTSD Revisits Painful Memories

PTSD is a special type of anxiety disorder that develops after a terrifying event in which serious physical or psychiatric harm occurred or was threatened, such as violent personal assaults, natural or human-caused disasters, accidents, or military combat. People with PTSD have recurring bad thoughts, dreams, and memories of this horrible ordeal. They also often have severe sleep problems, are easily startled, and feel emotionally detached from loved ones.

PTSD is very serious, and PTSD patients most often requires both medication and psychological treatments. Very often, the pain and the PTSD are so intermingled that they both need to improve simultaneously for either one to improve. The good news is that—as with the other psychological conditions—if treated appropriately, PTSD patients can and do improve.

TREATMENTS FOR DEPRESSION, ANXIETY DISORDER, AND PTSD

The good news is that all of these serious psychological conditions that can accompany chronic pain are treatable. Most patients do best with a combination of medication and psychological treatments.

If you think you may be suffering from depression, anxiety disorder, or PTSD, we strongly recommend that you be evaluated by a psychiatrist or psychologist, and if possible, one who is trained to work with chronic pain patients.

Medicines for Pschological Disorders

Most of the medications that are used to treat depression, anxiety disorder, and PTSD are the same. For almost every patient who suffers from one of these conditions, a doctor will be able to find a medication regimen that will work with minimal side effects. There are three types of medication: TCAs, serotonin-specific reuptake inhibiting medications, and selective serotonin and norepinephrine reuptake inhibitor (SSNRIs). We describe all of these medications in more depth in chapter 8.

Classes of Antidepressant Medications
TCAs
- Amitriptyline (Elavil)
- Nortriptyline (Pamelor)
- Desipramine (Norpramin)
- Doxepin (Sinequan)
- Imipramine (Tofranil)

SSRIs
- Fluoxetine (Prozac)
- Paroxetine (Paxil)
- Sertraline (Zoloft)
- Citalopram (Celexa)
- Escitalopram (Lexapro)

SSNRIs
- Venlafaxine (Effexor)
- Duloxetine (Cymbalta)
- Devenlafaxine (Prestiq)

Treatment Alert!

See a Pain Psychologist One of the most important elements of the treatment plan for chronic pain is to be evaluated and treated by a specialist referred to as a pain psychologist. Even if you are not found to have a psychological condition such as depression, anxiety, or PTSD, you can benefit greatly from learning some fairly simple psychological techniques.

Again, we want to reiterate how helpful these simple psychological techniques can be for most chronic pain patients. They do not involve looking into your childhood or your relationship with your mother; as you will see, they involve learning new ways of thinking about and reacting to your pain.

What's the Difference between a Psychiatrist and a Psychologist?

Even our relatives often don't understand this difference! A psychiatrist is a medical doctor (M.D.), and can prescribe medication. Most often nowadays, psychiatrists mostly specialize in medication management, choosing the right medicine(s) for you. A psychologist is a Ph.D. and cannot prescribe medication. But a psychologist is the one who is expert in assessing your condition and which types of psychological treatments may be best for you, and will train you on these techniques.

Nonmedication-Based Treatments for Chronic Pain
RELAXATION THERAPY REDUCES STRESS

You may be asking, "Relaxation? This is a form of psychological treatment?" Yes, it is. And it is a very useful type of "therapy" for many chronic pain patients. Relaxation therapy has a real and measurable effect on the underlying biology of pain, by reducing pain signals at the site of pain and your body's stress reaction. Although there are many different techniques to relaxation therapy, they all have the same goal: to minimize your body's response to stress. After reading chapter 17 on how stress has a direct, negative effect on your pain, you will understand why preventing the stress reaction can reap great and immediate benefits to you.

By reducing the amount of adrenaline (epinephrine) floating around your bloodstream, relaxation can minimize your pain flares associated with stress. Even a drop of adrenaline near damaged nerves or spastic muscles causes more pain. Damaged nerves and abnormally sensitive muscles become quite reactive to adrenaline, causing them to fire off more pain signals and go into more spasm, respectively. Relaxation teaches you ways to control the levels of adrenaline in your body, without any drugs. It's quite cool!

We're sure you've seen those TV shows demonstrating how Tibetan monks can do unbelievable things by controlling their bodies' "natural" reactions, such as body temperature or the ability to endure painful scenarios. You may not become a super-relaxer like one of those monks, but these simple relaxation techniques can help you gain more control over your body's reactions to stress.

The most common relaxation techniques taught to chronic pain patients include deep meditation, music- or sound-induced relaxation, mental imagery, and rhythmic, deep, visualized, or diaphragmatic breathing. Some patients have found good success with self-teaching relaxation via purchased CDs, tapes, and videos.

Regardless of the technique, most relaxation techniques involve the repetition of words, phrases, or movements. They also try to teach you to block out all other thoughts, similar to meditation.

Biofeedback aims to do similar things as relaxation, but with the use of a machine; we will discuss biofeedback shortly.

IMAGERY ALSO RELAXES THE MIND

Imagery is another favorite and easy technique taught to chronic pain patients. Simply, imagery helps you literally "escape to your favorite place." By helping you use your imagination to bring you there your body and mind immediately relax and make you feel good about life. If you are having trouble getting to your favorite place, you can use sensory aids, such as pictures, or smells, sounds, and tastes that remind you of the place. Some of the favorite places our patients visit are the Caribbean, a sporting event, the ski slopes, and family get-togethers. So, what's your favorite place? Maybe you have two or three! Go for a quick trip now.

BIOFEEDBACK HELPS YOU CONTROL YOUR STRESS REACTION

Biofeedback is a popular treatment used in treating chronic pain because it effectively teaches patients how to control their stress reaction, with no bad side effects. With biofeedback, you are hooked up to a device that can measure different bodily functions:

- Blood pressure
- Heart rate
- Skin temperature
- Sweat gland activity
- Muscle tension

The biofeedback machine allows you to obtain this information in real time, either by showing waves on a computer screen or by playing different pitches of noises. With training from a biofeedback practitioner, you will learn how to use relaxation techniques in your brain, body, and "mind" to alter these bodily functions.

A trained biofeedback therapist can make this learning process quicker and eventually teach you how to become aware of these internal bodily functions and control them without the machine. You may be saying to yourself, "There's no way I can be trained to do this, I'm not a master yogi!" However, it's important to realize that the vast majority of patients can be taught biofeedback and use it successfully.

Thus, biofeedback can help many chronic pain patients to recognize when their stress reaction is turned on, and then control the negative consequences of their pain.

Progressive Relaxation Means to Flex and Relax

Progressive relaxation is commonly taught by pain psychologists. This technique involves being taught how to flex specific muscles and hold the tension in those muscles for a minute or so, and then relaxing the muscles. Usually, the psychologist trains you to begin with your toes, and then your feet, and to slowly move up your body to your head, spending about one minute on each muscle group. With this technique, you should begin to notice when you are tensing your muscles and how to relax them. Eventually, you should also begin to notice when your muscles spontaneously become tense and how to relax them. When this happens, you are becoming aware of a possible stress reaction and hopefully are also learning how to prevent it from happening. (Hint: Before you start an actual progressive relaxation treatment session, you should find a comfortable position and remember to breathe.)

Find a Positive Support Group

As with many chronic medical conditions, many chronic pain patients find it helpful to join patient support groups to discuss shared experiences and learn from one another. Although these groups can often be very useful, we want to warn you that if they become more of a "gripe session" with folks just complaining and being negative, they can be harmful. Therefore, although we encourage you to find a chronic pain support group (whether it is specific to your pain condition or just a general chronic pain group), it is important that you find a group of chronic pain patients who are optimistic and helpful, while still being honest and truthful about their experiences. (Look in the Appendix for ways to contact organizations that can hook you up with an appropriate Support Group.)

COGNITIVE BEHAVIORAL THERAPY (CBT) HELPS YOU COPE

Cognitive behavioral therapy (CBT) has two important parts. The most important part is that you, the patient, need to understand how your thoughts and behaviors can greatly affect your pain, and just as importantly that you can have control over these thoughts and behaviors. In addition, CBT teaches certain coping-skill techniques that give you power over your pain.

You can learn many different techniques to help you gain control over how you react to and think about your pain. Most often, patients are trained in these techniques to determine which ones work best for them. CBT techniques can include relaxation therapies, which we just discussed. Another successful technique is cognitive restructuring. Cognitive restructuring helps you identify your negative pain-related thoughts. You then are asked to challenge the validity of these negative thoughts and replace them with ones that are more helpful to you. Although the technique may sound simple, many patients actually find it to be quite difficult. But when cognitive restructuring is done with a trained pain psychologist, most of our patients have told us that this technique was as important as the medications they used. After identifying your problem thoughts and behaviors, you are then taught to draw up plans on how and when to use your new thoughts and techniques.

Cognitive Restructuring Changes Your Thinking

Cognitive restructuring aims to identify unhelpful, irrational, or unachievable negative thoughts (described shortly) and replace them with more accurate ones. The cognitive restructuring theory believes that "faulty beliefs" generate negative emotions and behaviors, including stress, depression, anxiety, and social withdrawal. Thus, if we can rid ourselves of these negative thoughts that have no basis in reality, we can be rid of such negative emotions and behaviors and thereby improve our well-being and live with less pain.

Some of the more common faulty beliefs held by chronic pain patients are: "I can't deal with this pain anymore," "The more pain I feel, the more damage that's happening to my body," and "Because I can't do as much as I used to, I'm worthless." Though such thoughts may feel real, they need to be reexamined because they are simply not true. You have dealt with your pain before, so why can't you deal with it again? Think, "I have coped before, and now I will cope with my pain again." After reading this book, you should realize that the chronic pain you feel does not signify more damage in your body. As we describe in chapter 14, unlike acute pain usually caused by injury, the chronic pain you experience does not signal ongoing injury.

Once you realize that your chronic pain is not really causing damage to your body, you need to say to yourself, "The pain does not mean I am causing damage." At times, chronic pain patients begin to feel worthless because they cannot do as much as they could before they starting having chronic pain. However, you are still the same person inside, with the same experiences, knowledge, and relationships. Think, "I have lots to give to my family and my community, but now in new and different ways." And then go on and do it!

HYPNOSIS ACTUALLY WORKS FOR SOME

No, we're not recommending that you go to Las Vegas and plead with the hypnotist at Caesar's Palace for help! But truly, an experienced hypnotherapist can help some patients with chronic pain. Hypnosis has been successfully used to treat chronic pain in some patients for several decades. Although the mechanism by which hypnosis works is unknown, it is believed that hypnosis can alter the brain's functioning to reduce the perception of pain. Studies have actually demonstrated changes in brain activity in patients who are successfully hypnotized. Thus, although not commonly used, hypnosis can be of benefit to some people.

CONCLUSION: SEEK HELP FROM A PAIN PSYCHOLOGIST

Depression, anxiety disorders, and PTSD are the most common psychological conditions associated with chronic pain, regardless of type. Although common, not every patient will develop one of these conditions due to their chronic pain. However, if while reading this section you thought, "Hey, that sounds like me" please seek an evaluation from a psychiatrist or psychologist.

And remember, even if you are not depressed or anxious, or you do not have PTSD, you likely can still reap great rewards by learning proven, simple pain-relieving techniques from a pain psychologist.

CHAPTER 12

Multidisciplinary Pain Clinics Put It All Under One Roof

Many approaches are better than one.

An MPC is a place where all pain management health care providers work together as a unified team under one roof.

Patients benefit greatly from an environment in which different types of treatment providers can discuss each patient's care collaboratively on a regular basis.

- ✓ Physicians (neurologists, anesthesiologists, physiatrists, psychiatrists, etc.)
- ✓ Social workers, psychologists, and therapists
- ✓ Medication treatment
- ✓ Procedures (nerve block, trigger-point injection, spinal cord stimulation, etc.)
- ✓ Nonmedication treatments (biofeedback, hypnotherapy, physical therapy, acupuncture)

Questions to Ask a Pain or Headache Doctor

- What is your chronic pain (or headache) training?
- Where did you get your training on how to diagnose and treat [your condition]?
- How long did you train?

All pain specialists should have at least one year of specific fellowship training after residency training in multidisciplinary pain management.

Note that being "boarded" in pain medicine does not necessarily mean the doctor has had appropriate training. He or she may have had extensive training only in performing nerve blocks or inserting devices.

- Besides yourself, what other types of pain management health care providers do you work with?

All good pain specialists should be able to refer to and frequently work with other pain management providers whose expertise is different from theirs, such as neurologists, anesthesiologists, rehabilitation doctors, physical/occupational therapists, psychiatrists, psychologists, acupuncturists, biofeedback specialists, chiropractors, massage therapists, and so forth.

Make Sure It's The Real Deal!

You've probably seen a lot of signs reading "Pain Clinic," and perhaps even been to one or two. But not all pain clinics are created equal. In fact, many of the establishments claiming to be pain clinics are not qualified to treat you in the most effective way.

A real MPC has lots of different types of health care providers—physicians (anesthesiologists, neurologists), rehabilitation specialists (physiatrists), psychologists, physical therapists, occupational therapists, social workers, and so forth—all working closely together under one roof. Each professional has specific training and expertise in evaluating and treating all types of chronic pain, and all of the providers work together to give patients the best treatment for their condition. These are called *multidisciplinary* or *interdisciplinary pain clinics.*

BEWARE OF THE MONO-VISION PAIN CLINICS

Unfortunately, most places that call themselves "pain clinics" are not multidisciplinary at all. Most often, they are staffed by anesthesiologists who primarily perform nerve blocks and insert devices into patients' spinal cords (spinal cord stimulators and intrathecal medicine pumps), or they are staffed by a group of chiropractors or surgeons. Although there certainly is a role at times for all of these types of treatments, being evaluated for your pain by a mono-vision type of pain clinic that offers only one type of treatment will most likely not be in your best interest. Too many pain clinics typically will perform only the type of treatment that they know (and make money on), regardless of your type of pain.

If you go or are sent to one of these mono-vision pain clinics, beware. Remember the old saying, "When all you have is a hammer, everything looks like a nail." If simple treatments (medicine and physical/occupational therapy) are not working for you, find a true MPC (see appendix II).

CONCLUSION: MANY HEADS ARE BETTER THAN ONE

Because patients with chronic pain often need a mix of therapies, a multidisciplinary pain clinic is often the best place to receive treatment in a cohesive manner. At such a clinic, the appropriate treatments can be tailored to your specific needs and you can receive optimal treatment from trained pain specialists who work closely together for you.

CHAPTER 13

Caution: Surgery, Only When Necessary

(A Rare Event!)

Beware of quick fixes that will give you long-term disability issues.

the PRESCRIPTION for CHRONIC PAIN SURGERY

We placed this chapter on surgery as our last chapter in this part of the book for a reason:

Surgery is rarely an option for chronic pain patients. Too often, especially in our society of "quick fixes," patients hope that their pain can be quickly cured by surgery. Well, let us warn you that we have seen many more patients made worse by having surgery for their pain condition than were made better. Thus, surgery should be reserved for only infrequent and specific pain conditions.

Rare Conditions That Warrant Surgery

Of course, there are reasons to have surgery for your chronic pain, but they are infrequent and specific. For instance, surgery is definitely warranted if you have back pain caused by an extruded disc (a piece of disc has broken off and is floating in your spinal canal) and/or a severe bulging disc that is causing you to also have foot/leg weakness or bowel or bladder incontinence. It is also warranted if you have severe debilitating knee or hip osteoarthritis (OA) that other, more conservative treatments have failed to cure, if you have carpal tunnel syndrome that doesn't respond to many of the nonsurgical treatments, or if you have a tumor on a nerve causing you neuropathic (nerve injury) pain. Really, that's about it!

Inappropriate Recommendations for Surgery

After managing patients with chronic pain for a number of years, we have come to realize that protecting our patients from potentially dangerous treatments is just as important as finding the appropriate treatments for them. We have seen too much damage done to our patients who listened to uneducated surgeons and agreed to have surgery for many pain conditions, only to be made worse by the surgery. And often, to make the situation worse, the surgeon then blames the patient for not getting better. (Believe it or not, this happens all the time!)

BACK SURGERY ONLY MAKES IT WORSE

There is no indication for back surgery unless the patient meets the criteria listed in the sidebar. This warning goes out to people contemplating their first back surgery, or to "repeat offenders" who keep having back surgery because earlier surgeries have failed. Back surgery is probably one of the most unnecessarily performed surgeries in the United States. And again, what makes this situation even sadder is that many patients are made worse by the surgery.

SINUS SURGERY FOR "CHRONIC SINUS HEADACHE"

It is still not scientifically proven that there is such a thing as "chronic sinus headache"; one study demonstrated that most patients who are told they have "sinus headaches" actually have migraines or tension-type headaches. Here, too, many patients who undergo surgery are made worse by the damage and scarring done by the surgery.

Select Conditions That Warrant Surgery

- Low back pain due to severe disc disease only when associated with weakness or bowel/bladder dysfunction
- OA of the knee or hip, only with severe pain and disability, having failed other treatments
- Carpal tunnel syndrome, only when there is intractable pain, weakness, and/or loss of sensation
- Presence of tumors pressing on nerves

213

CARPAL TUNNEL SYNDROME

Yes, we did just recommend surgery for the appropriate patient. However, many people have surgery for carpal tunnel either don't actually have the condition or could have done fine (or even better) without surgery.

REMOVING "SCAR TISSUE"

We have seen patients get this surgery in an attempt to resolve back pain, neck pain, pelvic pain, and other forms of pain. Remember: When you remove scar tissue, you can rip the underlying healthy tissue, and the scar tissue will just grow back! This surgery usually exacerbates the pain.

CUTTING OFF A NEUROMA

If you have a neuroma (an abnormal bundle of nerves) removed, you will experience pain relief. However, over several months, the nerve will attempt to grow where it was cut, and you will develop another new neuroma that may be more difficult to treat.

HYSTERECTOMY FOR MENSTRUAL MIGRAINES

This is one of the scariest operations, and we have seen it done! First, it's typically just plain stupid. Second, it doesn't work! One of the saddest situations we have seen involves young women who have had their uterus and ovaries removed who still have migraines and now cannot have children. Although sometimes removing the ovaries can reduce or eliminate menstrual migraine, most women still will get other migraines. So they now not only still have migraines, they are infertile.

Avoid "Exploratory" Surgery

Among the many surgeries to avoid, there is one in particular that far too many pain patients undergo: exploratory surgery. This term generally describes surgery that is performed to find the source of pain and in most cases fails to do so. If a doctor tells you he or she wants to perform exploratory surgery, we can offer one piece of advice: Consider running away from that doctor!

The sad fact is that when exploratory surgery is performed to "find the source of pain," not only will the reason for the pain likely remain a mystery, but also your pain may worsen after the operation.

CONCLUSION: NO QUICK FIX FOR CHRONIC PAIN

Unfortunately, a quick-fix surgery is rarely the answer for most patients with chronic pain, although you can likely find a surgeon who is willing to participate. Compounding the problem is the fact that most doctors, especially surgeons, are not appropriately trained in diagnosing and treating most chronic pain conditions, and insurance companies are more likely to reimburse you for surgery rather than for a visit to a multidisciplinary pain clinic or for participation in a physical therapy program. Here, it is important to remember: You can't simply take what looks like the easy way out. If the solution to your pain looks too good to be true, it probably is. Proper pain management takes effort from you and your physician, but don't give up! Remember: You can do it!

PART 3

Understanding Your Pain

CHAPTER 14

What Is Pain? Why Do We Experience It?

Understand the new thinking behind chronic pain.

Let Us Ask You: What Is Pain?

It's hard to come up with a precise definition, isn't it? Well, you're not alone. Brilliant doctors, scientists, and even philosophers have had great difficulty too. Pain has defied scientific definition for a long time. Sir Thomas Lewis, one of the premier British medical scientists of the twentieth century, wrote, "I am so far from being able satisfactorily to define pain ... that the attempt could serve no useful purpose." And Henry Ward Beecher, regarded by many as the greatest American clerical orator of his century, stated in 1859: "...philosophers and scientists have none of them succeeded in defining pain."

In 1973, a group of pain experts from around the world met near Seattle to discuss clinical and scientific issues in pain research and patient care. One of the most important and challenging tasks on the agenda for this group of wise men and women was to reach an agreed-upon definition of pain. This group later evolved into the prestigious International Association for the Study of Pain (IASP), which now has more than 6,500 members from more than 100 countries. After much spirited debate and discussion, the IASP members came up with the following definition in 1973:

The Definition Of Pain

"Pain is an unpleasant sensory and emotional experience associated with actual or potential tissue damage or described in terms of such damage."

UNDERSTANDING THE DEFINITION OF PAIN

This definition of pain has withstood several decades of scrutiny and still remains the most accepted and most widely used definition of pain today. Several very important concepts are hidden within this seemingly simple, one-sentence definition of pain.

"Unpleasant Sensory and Emotional Experience"

Unlike our other senses—sight, hearing, smell, taste, and touch—the sensation of pain is always associated with a distinctly unpleasant emotion. Just think of your past painful experiences—were any of them pleasant? (We hope not, or then you'd have another problem!)

"Actual or Potential Tissue Damage"

When you were asked to think of prior experiences that resulted in pain, you most likely thought of activities that caused an injury to your body, such as a cut, a bruise, a muscle sprain or strain, or perhaps a broken bone. Indeed, all of these would cause you to feel something you would call "pain."

Now let's remember the time you put your hand on that steaming hot cup of coffee and had to quickly put the cup down on the table. Most likely, you didn't burn yourself (and hence experienced no injury), but it still hurt like heck. It felt like you could have done some damage, right? This type of pain is an example of "potential" bodily damage, meaning that if you had not felt the burning pain and put the cup on the table, you likely would have damaged your hand with a burn.

This is an example of what we call *potential tissue injury*. And it hurts just like actual tissue damage, but no actual injury occurs.

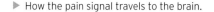

▶ How the pain signal travels to the brain.

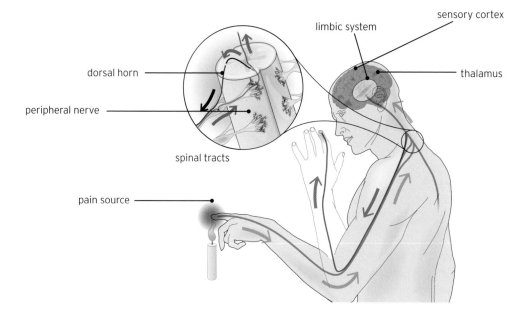

The Difference Between Acute and Chronic Pain

You might ask yourself: Why make a distinction between acute pain and chronic pain? They both hurt, don't they? It is important to distinguish between these types of pain because, although they have much in common, their differences have a significant impact on how doctors diagnosis and treat you. **Although the role of pain is very helpful when acute, it is completely inappropriate and counterproductive when chronic.**

Acute pain begins following any injury, which can be minor, such as stubbing your toe, or major, such as pain associated with surgery or a heart attack. Whether minor or major damage happens, after you injure yourself a series of bodily events occurs. Once the damage or danger is no longer present, you stop feeling pain.

CHRONIC PAIN OCCURS AFTER THE HURT HAS HEALED

Chronic pain is quite different. Unfortunately, believe it or not, there is no widely accepted simple definition of chronic pain. Chronic pain is defined not only by its time course—that is, the longevity of the pain following the acute injury—but more importantly by the determination that the healing process itself has been completed. Patients with chronic pain report that their pain is worse than their prior experience with acute pain. They say that chronic pain is tiring, frustrating, and never-ending. Acute pain is easier to deal with, physically and psychologically, because you know that it will eventually go away. In the case of chronic pain, however, there appears to be no end in sight. Now that hurts.

The Tsunami Of Chronic Pain

As stated in the IASP's definition of pain, pain is both a sensation and an emotion. However, pain is even more complex than that description implies. When we look at the individual pain sufferer (you) and how the pain has affected your life, we can see that pain has a large rippling effect, like a pebble thrown onto the surface of still water. Or perhaps a better image is one of multiple small waves that, when added together, cause a powerful and destructive tsunami.

The tsunami of waves causes upheaval and stress in the lives of you and those around you, such as workplace changes, complications in insurance, and legal and workers' compensation. All of these negative and very stressful life events build and build, eventually causing "the tsunami of chronic pain." You often feel crushed and overwhelmed by these problems. It seems like no matter where you look and no matter what time of day it is, you are faced with pain and all the additional stress it causes. You just want to get the heck away!

221

Why Do We Experience Pain?

Put simply, pain makes us remember how we injured ourselves and teaches us not to do it again. Pain causes a strong memory to imprint in our brains so that we avoid similar dangerous activities in the future. Pain also forces us to protect an injured body part so that we don't cause further injury. If we walk on a broken foot, we feel more pain, so we stop doing it, thus preventing further damage. Like it or not, you need to experience pain to survive. Just as hunger and thirst are basic drives that we need to survive, we need the sensation of pain to survive. And just as hunger and thirst are instinctual experiences that develop in our brains, so does pain. Remember: Pain alerts us to real or potential injury.

Indeed, on top of the horrible pain and emotions you feel inside, other unwelcome "waves" from the tsunami arrive as impediments in your quest to find relief. It is important that both you and your pain doctor evaluate how these waves affect you. In the following sections, we will outline some of the complications (waves) and how best to manage them.

WAVE 1: TOO MUCH LOVE FROM FRIENDS AND FAMILY

How can your family or friends show too much affection? Through excessive love and caring, they may actually be making your overall situation worse. For instance, your loving spouse may be doing all your household chores because he or she does not want you to feel more pain. A loved one may express his or her concern by not wanting you to move (because it worsens your pain). But by doing all your chores and activities, your loved one may be inadvertently worsening your condition. Trying to protect you from moving your body may cause some of the problems we talked about earlier to arise (e.g., muscle weakening and spasm, etc.).

Similarly, in an attempt to help you limit your activity, friends may refrain from including you in opportunities for social interaction, which can isolate you and cause or worsen depression. This misplaced love can become a big wave in the growing tsunami of chronic pain.

WAVE 2: THE NEGATIVE EFFECTS ON YOUR FAMILY

As though it wasn't bad enough already, the tsunami can become even more powerful. Very often, your role in the family is dramatically altered. You may not be able to work and support your family. You may not be able to care for your younger, older, or sick family members. Quite often, therefore, the pain felt by one family member is in effect "felt" by the entire family.

WAVE 3: LOSS OF SELF-ESTEEM

Along with your inability to perform your normal tasks comes a loss of self-esteem. You lose the pride that comes with the ability to help and support people, including yourself. It may feel as though you lose your sense of place in this world. This loss is a giant wave, adding power to the tsunami.

WAVE 4: THE INSURANCE, LEGAL, AND WORKERS' COMPENSATION SYSTEMS

Do you have a lawsuit or workers' compensation claim related to your pain? If so, you are adding another huge wave to the tsunami. Even though the vast majority of chronic pain patients who are involved in a lawsuit or workers' compensation case have justifiable complaints and are not looking for a large settlement, it is likely they are not being treated nicely by the third party involved.

Another sad fact (we warned you there were lots of these) is that the legal and workers' compensation systems still put up barriers for the person in chronic pain. **More often than not, they treat you as though you are guilty until proven innocent.** Having to work your way through the insurance, legal, and workers' compensation systems is unbelievably frustrating and time-consuming. And having to do so only adds further unneeded stress (of the psychological type) to your horrible situation.

Believe it or not, if you are in such a situation, it is equally as important to find an experienced, kind, and ethical lawyer as it is to find a good doctor. A good lawyer can dramatically improve the quality of life of a person in pain; it is worth taking your time to find the right person to serve you.

It is also important to beware of doctors who automatically view people in pain as "bad" if they have ongoing lawsuits and workers' compensation issues. On the other hand, you should be equally wary of doctors who have been recommended by lawyers or colleagues who only see patients with legal or workers' compensation issues—they may not have your best interest (i.e., getting better!) at heart. If either of these scenarios is the case, find yourself another doctor.

All Pain Is Real

You, your family, and your doctors must realize that a lot of people experience pain, especially chronic pain, without having any obvious bodily damage or ongoing potential tissue damage. In fact, very often, chronic pain patients have completely normal physical examinations and laboratory tests. How can that be?

With many types of chronic pain, the usual tests do not reveal anything wrong or abnormal in the body to explain why the person is experiencing pain. But if you have chronic pain and all your lab tests are "normal," something abnormal is

The Importance of a Doctor Who Believes You

Let me tell you a personal story that I hold dear and that still rings true. When I, Dr. Galer, was at the University of Washington Pain Clinic, I opened a clinic for patients suffering from a fairly uncommon chronic pain condition, Reflex Sympathetic Dystrophy (now called CRPS). There, I worked with a pain psychologist and a physical therapist, and together we cared for these patients for several years. When I decided to leave Seattle, the patients requested a group session with me. I thought I was going to walk into a gripe session, because for many of these patients, though they made tremendous gains, it took me awhile to find the right mixture of therapies to offer them some pain relief. What I heard from every single one of them was something like the following: "Dr. Galer, more important than the pain relief you gave me was something no other doctor could give me. You listened to me and believed that I had real pain. And telling me that I wasn't crazy or a crock was the most important thing you gave me." Well, that was more than ten years ago, and their voices still speak loudly to me today.

still occurring in your body, likely in your nervous system or muscles. A lack of examination findings does not imply that the problem is "in your head" (psychological). Rather, it implies that your underlying problem causing your pain cannot be detected by current assessment techniques doctors have available to them today. The tests today are simply not good enough to detect most nervous system activity—normal or abnormal. Remember, before the advent of MRI machines, many patients were misdiagnosed because doctors couldn't actually see where the problem was and all the older radiology types of tests were normal. Still, either the medical testing equipment today is not sensitive enough to detect the abnormality in your body, or we, the medical community, are still too ignorant to know what to measure and look for.

Even today, doctors frequently tell their chronic pain patients that it's all in their head and there's nothing they can do. However, what you and your doctors must realize is that all tests have their limits, especially tests assessing pain. It is very likely that no laboratory test will ever be able to find the source in most persons suffering with chronic pain.

TEACHING HUMILITY TO DOCTORS

Unfortunately, many doctors need to practice a bit of humility and realize that there is still much to be learned about pain. Too often, we doctors make lots of assumptions based on prior (incorrect) teachings or are afraid to admit we don't know something. Here are some instances when the medical profession was just plain wrong and too many patients suffered because of it. **In medical school, we were taught that more than 90 percent of what we were learning would be found to be incorrect or only partially true within 10 years!**

Migraines: A Mental Problem? No!

Did you realize that migraines were once believed to be a psychiatric problem? Believe it or not, only in the past decade or so have medical schools treated migraine headaches as having a biological cause. Why?

- Physical examinations by doctors were normal.
- Laboratory tests were normal.
- Migraine often occurred in the setting of stress.
- Migraine occurred most frequently in women.

You may remember that "way back when," many conditions occurring in women were not taken seriously or believed to by due to "hysteria." Unfortunately, this bias still affects some areas of medicine.

Luckily, migraines are now finally accepted to be a real medical disease. How did mainstream doctors see the light? In the 1990s, two important events happened. First, a patient serendipitously had a migraine attack during a magnetic resonance imaging scan, which showed "real changes in the brain." Second, around the same time, researchers discovered a new class of migraine-specific drugs (triptans) that target a specific brain chemical that stops these headaches. These advances in science have significantly helped our efforts to diagnose and treat patients with migraines.

When Phantom Pain Didn't Exist

Another example of our profession's ignorance and bad judgment regarding a medical condition concerns phantom pain. Phantom pain is when a person complains of chronic pain in an arm or leg (or any body part) that has been amputated. For centuries, these persons in pain were considered psychologically disturbed. The esteemed medical community believed they were mourning and grieving for their lost body parts. These poor suffering patients were actually institutionalized in psychiatric wards! We now have evidence that phantom pain is most likely a brain disorder; following amputation, changes are clearly seen in certain brain regions controlling the amputated limb's sensory and motor functions. Luckily, nowadays soldiers coming back from Iraq and Afghanistan who suffer traumatic amputations and develop phantom limb pain will more likely be properly treated.

Today's Invisible Sufferers

Despite all the progress we have made, we still live in the Dark Ages when it comes to chronic pain. Even today, sufferers of chronic pain can feel discredited and isolated. For example, those with Reflex Sympathetic Dystrophy/ Complex Regional Pain Syndrome (RSD/CRPS, see chapter 4) are being denied treatment and health benefits because their pain is still believed to be psychogenic. **Indeed, even today, chronic pain patients are often given the wrong treatment or denied insurance benefits because some uneducated doctor is blinded by his or her lack of education and lack of humility.** Now you see why you need to be armed with proper knowledge to make sure this doesn't happen to you.

Pain Alert!

It's Not in Your Head
Too often, when tests are normal and your doctor cannot find a reason why you have chronic pain, the doctor wrongly assumes your pain is psychological. The doctor is wrong, wrong, wrong!

Break the Vicious Cycle of Chronic Pain

The Vicious Cycle of Chronic Pain (VCCP) probably occurs in far more than 90 percent of people with chronic pain, as a natural response to the condition. The problem is that the VCCP is bad, very bad—it not only keeps you in pain, but also usually causes your state to worsen. What is the VCCP? Let's discuss its primary components.

When someone with chronic pain moves the painful body part, he or she typically experiences an increase in pain. This is because the patient has not been using the body part normally, resulting in:

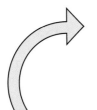

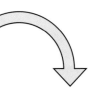

- Muscle tightness and muscle spasm
- Ligament and tendon shortening and tightening

- The experience of increased pain with movement then results in fear—fear of more damage being done to the already painful body part. This is because, as far as the person's brain is concerned, all pain automatically means "injury."

- From these events, more disuse results, leading to:
  - More loss of muscle, tendon, and ligament elasticity (tightening)
  - More muscle atrophy, weakness, and spasm

- Pain and fear then automatically cause the stress reaction to be turned on (see chapter 17).

- Pain, fear, and the stress reaction then result in further guarding and protection of the painful body part and even less movement of it.

▶ And thus, the cycle starts again.

THE BRAIN UNDER STRESS MAKES PAIN WORSE

Now do you see why we call it the Vicious Cycle of Chronic Pain? In the presence of chronic pain, the discomfort you feel with each movement of your body part is not due to additional damage, but rather is the result of the development of tight muscles, tendons, and ligaments, and the anxiety you feel from fear. If you are not reassured by your health care providers that this pain is not causing you more injury, it is only natural for you to believe that more damage is being done with every sharp pain you experience during movement. Your brain will then automatically turn on the stress reaction, which will tell you to stop moving.

CONCLUSION: FIND THE TREATMENT YOU DESERVE!

If your doctor, insurance company, or lawyer tells you the pain is all in your head, based only on the fact that your lab tests and examinations are normal, please (let us be brutally honest—you must) find an educated and trained pain physician to properly assess and treat you. For many chronic pain patients, one of the most important things a doctor can do is to validate their pain by saying, "Yes, the pain is real. Yes, you are suffering from the pain. Yes, I will try to treat your pain, even if I cannot identify the cause. It is not in your head—I believe you."

Pain Alert!

Get Educated and Get Moving! Unfortunately, the terrible mistake of fearing movement is often reinforced by ill-advised health care providers who say "If it hurts, don't do it." With this approach, more guarding and protection and lack of appropriate movement occur, resulting in even more musculoskeletal changes, more pain, and the indefinite perpetuation of the VCCP. For this reason, it is crucial that you educate yourself (as you are doing by reading this!) and be reassured that the pain you feel with activity and physical therapy will not be harmful and is a necessary part of treatment.

CHAPTER 15

A Brief Tour of the Nervous System

Understand the anatomy of how your body creates pain.

Don't Skip These Pages!

We know you want to turn the page (or flick your e-reader finger), but don't!

The purpose of this section is not to turn you off, but to turn you on to how your body creates the perception of pain. Trust us—it's important to learn about your nervous system so that you can better understand your pain, so read on! Here, we will follow your pain signal from its birth in the peripheral nervous system, into your spinal cord, and finally up to your brain. Okay! Let's start the lesson.

PERIPHERAL AND CENTRAL NERVOUS SYSTEMS

The nervous system is subdivided into two parts: the peripheral nervous system and the central nervous system. The peripheral nervous system consists of all of the nerves in your skin, muscles, and organs that travel to and from the spinal cord. Your spinal cord and brain make up your central nervous system. Simple, right?

▼ Normal pain signal's travel

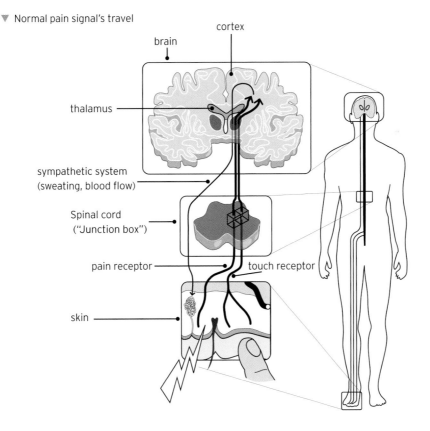

cortex

brain

thalamus

sympathetic system
(sweating, blood flow)

Spinal cord
("Junction box")

pain receptor   touch receptor

skin

The Role of the Peripheral Nervous System in Pain

To repeat: Your peripheral nervous system consists of all of the nerves in your skin, muscles, and organs that travel to and from the spinal cord. The nerves of the peripheral nervous system are made up of two basic types based on what they do: your motor nerves and your sensory nerves. The motor nerves go from the spinal cord and travel to your muscles. When activated, these motor nerves cause your muscles to move (by either contracting or extending the muscle).

Your sensory nerves are more important than the motor nerves with regard to pain (no surprise). Sensory nerves, as their name implies, relay information about different sensations you may be feeling. Sensory nerves are further divided based on their size: large sensory peripheral nerves and small sensory peripheral nerves.

LARGE NERVES SENSE VIBRATIONS

Have you ever had a doctor put a tuning fork on your toe or finger? Why would the doctor do that? This is how your doctor tests how well your large peripheral sensory nerves are working. Large peripheral sensory nerves detect information about vibrations. To test how your large sensory nerves are working, a doctor will hit a tuning fork, causing it to vibrate, and then place it on your body parts, usually your large toe, and ask you when you stop feeling it vibrate. In addition, these large nerve fibers are the ones that help you (and your brain) figure out where your body parts are in space (this is called *proprioception*). For instance, close your eyes and put your hand above your head. If your large peripheral sensory nerves are working normally, you knew that your hand was above your head without looking. However, if these nerves are not working correctly, you would have no idea where your arm was. This can happen in people who develop neuropathy (see chapter 4). People with large-fiber neuropathy are not able to tell where their feet are when they are walking in the dark, and may therefore feel off-balance, causing them to trip or fall.

SMALL NERVES SENSE PAIN AND TEMPERATURE

Now let's find out about your small sensory nerves, which are more important when it comes to pain. These nerves will be stimulated, for example, by poking the skin with a pin. Small sensory nerve fibers detect this stimulation and send this painful information from your body to your spinal cord. These nerves can also detect temperature information. That's why a doctor may sometimes put a cold or hot object on your skin, to test how well these small peripheral nerves are working.

Two things can happen when the small sensory nerves are damaged. Sometimes a patient will lose his or her ability to feel pain and temperature in the skin area of that nerve. These people need to be careful because they may hurt themselves without realizing they are doing so. For example, they may burn themselves from scalding hot bath water and not feel it. Or they can be walking with a pebble in their shoe and not notice it.

In other patients, the opposite can happen. When these small sensory nerves get damaged or inflamed, they can actually become hyperactive and hypersensitive. If this is the case, small sensory nerves cause pain when there's really no reason to feel it. When this happens, the small sensory nerves short-circuit, like a frayed electrical wire, and constantly send pain signals to the spinal cord and brain.

How Your Nerves Talk to Each Other

As you will see, we don't have one big nerve that travels from our skin or muscles all the way up to our brain. Multiple nerves are connected along the way. These nerves need to talk to one another for information to be passed along from one to another. Nerves communicate with one another in two major ways: electrically and chemically.

ELECTRIC AVENUE

A nerve is like an electric cable, with the electric current starting at one end of the nerve and traveling to the other end. The electric cable portion of the nerve is called the *axon*. Once the current starts in one end of the axon, it will automatically travel to the other end.

However, when this electric current reaches the end of the first nerve (let's call this *Nerve A*), a critical thing happens. The receiving nerve (*Nerve B*) must decide whether this electrical information is worthy of continuing the message along its axon, bringing it closer to the brain. So, even if the nerve signal reaches the space between two connected nerves (called the *synapse*) there is no guarantee that the signal will automatically move into the next nerve.

In the simplest case, the electric current itself determines whether the signal in question is passed along to the next nerve. If there is enough electric energy, the green light is given and the electrical information is simply transferred from one nerve to the next nerve (Nerve A to Nerve B). However, in many cases, another factor will determine whether the signal moves along: chemical communication.

CHEMICALS MODULATE ELECTRIC SIGNALS

Chemicals called *neurotransmitters* modulate electric communication along the nerves. Neurotransmitters are produced in the first nerve (Nerve A) when the current reaches the end of its axon. Nerve A's neurotransmitters are then released into the space (the synapse) between Nerve A and Nerve B. Attached to the beginning of Nerve B (the side facing the synapse) are receptors, sort of like baseball gloves whose sole purpose is to catch specific neurotransmitters from Nerve A. The system works like a lock and key—when the appropriate neurotransmitter (the key) binds to the receptor (the lock) it causes the door to unlock. When the receptor is unlocked the information from Nerve A is transferred to Nerve B.

▼ Neurotransmitter communication

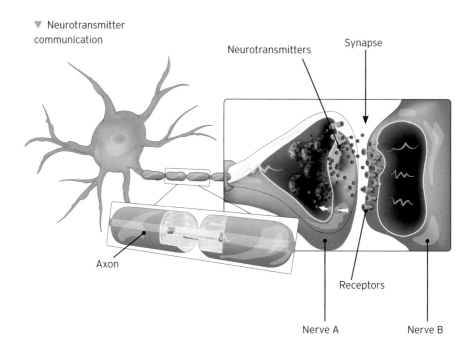

Neurotransmitters

Synapse

Axon

Receptors

Nerve A

Nerve B

However, when Nerve A's neurotransmitter key finds Nerve B's receptor lock, it does not automatically mean that the "door will open," allowing information to be passed into Nerve B. Some neurotransmitters will open the lock and pass the signal to Nerve B, a process called *excitation*. However, other neurotransmitters will lock the door even tighter and stop the information from being transferred into Nerve B, a process called *inhibition*.

Got it? You might need to read this a couple of times, but once you do, it's pretty cool! Now read on because, like most things in life, it ain't that simple. Continue to the next section to see how things can get even cooler!

The "Pain Gate" in Your Spinal Cord

So, now Nerve A's chemical neurotransmitter key is inside Nerve B's receptor lock. If the neurotransmitter can manage to unlock the receptor, the information will continue on toward the spinal cord. Let's look at the big picture.

Remember the large peripheral nerves? They also help to move the pain signal along. Both the large and small peripheral nerves (from the skin or muscles) converge together onto the spinal cord, Nerve B. In other words, the pain nerve in the spinal cord (Nerve B) receives information from both the large (motor and proprioception) peripheral nerves and the small (pain and temperature) peripheral nerves. How do these two types of nerves work together?

THE GATE CONTROL THEORY

In 1965, to explain how the pain nerve in the spinal cord (Nerve B) uses the information from both the large and small nerves, two pain scientist "gods," Patrick Wall and Ronald Melzack, devised the Gate Control Theory. The Gate Control Theory states that, like an old-time scale, Nerve B in the spinal cord weighs all of the information it receives from the large and small sensory nerves. The amount of (+) pain information (electrical and chemical) coming from the small nerves is weighed against the (-) pain information (electrical and chemical) being sent by the large nerves; in other words, the information from the small peripheral nerves is "excitatory" and the information from the large peripheral nerves is "inhibitory." The spinal sensory nerve in the spinal cord (Nerve B) is continuously adding all of the (+)s and (-)s that it is receiving. The role of the spinal cord nerve is basically that of "gatekeeper": Should it let the pain signal pass or should it stop it from proceeding? If you're a Monty Python fan, it's like the Black Knight in *Monty Python and The Holy Grail*!

If there are more (+)s than (-)s, the pain information is allowed to pass into the spinal cord sensory Nerve B and continue on to the next nerve in the brain. If the (-)s outweigh the (+)s, the pain signal is stopped and does not continue up the spinal cord to the brain. Makes sense, right? **This process of adding and subtracting pain signals in the spinal cord from the small and large nerve fibers became known as the *Gate Control Theory*.**

Since 1965, this theory has gained an overwhelming amount of supporting evidence regarding what happens to the pain signal, and is generally accepted by pain scientists and physicians worldwide.

▼ Gate control theory

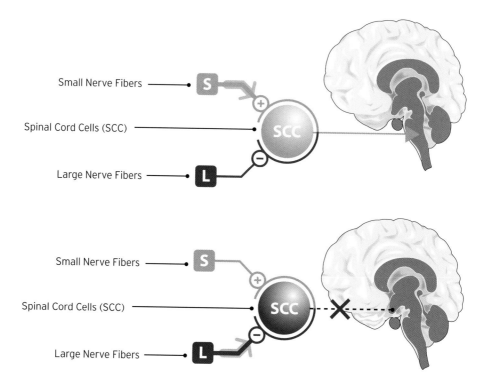

Your Most Important Organ: The Brain

After the Gate Control Theory became widely accepted, a crucial new scientific finding was made: Your brain plays a major role in controlling your pain. **How you are feeling or what you are thinking about your pain has a direct impact on what happens to the pain signal in the spinal cord, and thus has a huge effect on how much pain you feel!**

FROM THE SPINAL CORD TO THE BRAIN AND BACK

Your brain has a direct connection to Nerve B in your spinal cord. Your brain sends nerves directly into the same pain region of the spinal cord as do your small and large peripheral nerves. And wouldn't you know it, your brain can also send both excitatory (+) pain signals and inhibitory (-) pain signals. The brain then also has a vote as to whether the pain signal will continue up to it or stop in the spinal cord. In other words, your brain modulates all of your pain signals even before the pain signals reach it. **Input from your brain can either amplify (increase) the pain signal or dampen (decrease) the pain signal as it leaves the spinal cord on its way up to the brain.** Now that's fascinating!

We will discuss this in more depth later in this chapter. For now, let's assume that the pain signal has been given the green light at the spinal cord and the pain information has been transferred to Nerve B. What happens next? Once in the spinal cord's Nerve B (called the *spinothalamic nerve tract*), the pain signal simply travels up to the brain. The spinal cord acts as a conduit, a simple electric cable, transferring the pain signal from the peripheral nervous system, along the spinothalamic tract, and into the brain.

Once in the brain, the pain signal travels to an area called the *thalamus*. The thalamus is a structure in the middle of the brain that acts like a big city train station. Here, nerve signals coming from all parts of your body arrive to make their first connection in the brain. When the pain signal arrives here, it can be directed to multiple brain areas at the same time, including areas responsible for the sensation, emotion, and memories associated with pain. The signal can also be sent to motor areas of the brain, responsible for your movement response to the pain. The brain will not only "perceive" or feel your pain, but also trigger an action plan as to how you should respond, with regard to your behavior, your emotions, and your physical movements.

HOW YOUR BRAIN RESPONDS TO PAIN

First, let's learn a little about how the brain works. Most scientists believe it is the most complex machine ever created. Indeed, without our brain we would not perceive any pain (truly, we couldn't perceive anything at all). The sensations and emotions of pain occur due to complex interactions among many different parts of the brain.

As we discussed earlier, after the pain signal travels from the peripheral nervous system through the spinal cord and finally reaches the brain, the signal spreads rapidly to many different regions of the brain. The brain is a bundle of infinite systems that are constantly talking to and working with each other. No one brain region can work by itself; to work at its highest potential, each region needs to be in constant communication with many other areas in the brain.

Pain processing is no exception. Many regions of the brain continually communicate to determine the cause of the pain and the best response to the pain you are feeling. Once received by the brain, the pain signal can take a number of paths

How pain works in the brain ▼

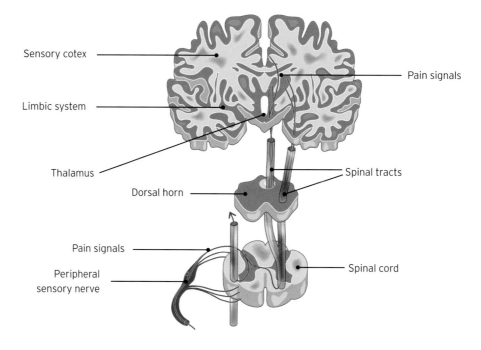

to produce different responses. However, regardless of the particular path, the end result must always be a unified, integrated, and cohesive response. In other words, all the parts of your brain need to work together to form a response that makes sense and helps you cope with your current situation. (For instance, after being mangled by a lion, you don't want to be fearful and teary-eyed and find yourself running directly into the lion's mouth!)

Let's take a closer look at these different activities and the brain regions that are involved.

The Brain and the Sensation of Pain

As we just discussed, once the pain signal reaches your brain, it goes to an area called the *thalamus*. The thalamus lies deep within the middle of your brain and is a structure where many different types of sensations, such as vision, hearing, and smell, all make connections. For the sensation of pain, after visiting the thalamus the pain signal travels to the sensory cortex (the worm-like covering of the brain). The sensory cortex has many different areas, each one dedicated to different senses and body regions.

The sensory cortex is thought to play important roles in the perception of pain. First, it determines the pain's intensity (i.e., the pain signal's strength) and the location of the pain (e.g., arm, leg, or back). The sensory cortex then labels the pain as being good (like exercise pain) or bad (as in a possible bodily injury). It is very important for your brain to make this distinction so that it knows what to do next. Should you cry and pull your hand away (e.g., if your hand is touching a hot teapot), or should you ignore the pain and keep focusing on your running (e.g., when you are running a marathon)? This labeling of the pain as good or bad is critical in chronic pain, as you will see later in this chapter.

The Brain and the Emotion of Pain

As you now know, pain is always associated with a negative emotional response, even when you're exercising. It shouldn't feel good (unless you're a masochist!). So, what part of the brain is responsible for this emotional response? This is a question that continues to puzzle neuroscientists and philosophers alike. Currently, scientists seem to think that a region in the brain called the *limbic system* may be necessary for us to experience both good and bad emotions. Science has also shown, in human brain scan studies, that the pain signal always goes to the limbic system. In fact, there is evidence that in some types of pain, the pain signal can go directly from the spinal cord to the limbic system without passing through the thalamus. Additionally, the limbic system, including the amygdala, stores important memories, including ones crucial to your survival—so, you can see why connections to the pain signal would be helpful.

The Brain's Autonomic Nervous System and Pain

The autonomic nervous system (ANS) is composed of several structures within the brain that are also crucial for survival. The ANS, like the limbic system, is an ancient part of the brain (all animals, no matter how intelligent, have this part of the brain) that controls your blood flow, heart rhythm, and breathing rate. The ANS is connected to other brain areas and to other organs in the body, which work together to create and implement the stress reaction—the "fight or flight" reaction.

Many of the ANS brain regions are directly involved with pain and its emotions. These regions include many parts of the limbic system, such as the anterior cingulate cortex, amygdala, periaqueductal gray, and hypothalamus. The ANS also has connections to the peripheral nerves that go to your skin, muscles, blood vessels, and pupils. You will see further in this chapter how all of these brain and body parts work together to make the stress reaction occur automatically.

The Brain's Motor System and Pain

As you have already learned, we have pain to warn us that potential injury is about to occur or bodily damage has already taken place. Therefore, it makes sense that pain is not an end unto itself, but rather must result in an action, a motor response, to keep us alive. The motor system in the brain consists of the motor cortex, which connects to muscles by sending nerves down our spinal cord and then to our peripheral motor nerves, which then connect to our muscles. Other brain areas are also involved in planning and coordinating your movements, such as the premotor cortex, supplementary motor area, posterior parietal cortex, and cerebellum.

So, now you are beginning to see all the activity that happens behind the scenes in your brain the split second you begin to feel pain—and even before you actually feel it.

PAIN MODULATION IN THE BRAIN

You'll note that this section is relatively long compared to the others. We've written somewhat more on brain modulation because you can actually use this natural inborn ability to help with your pain (and also because we've always found this topic fascinating!).

Let's start with an example of what is meant by *pain modulation*. When a baby falls down, she cries. But when the baby's mother picks her up and holds her, the crying soon ends. Do you think this is because the baby was not really feeling pain, but just wanted attention? Maybe, but that's unlikely.

Believe it or not, the mother's picking up the baby and holding her most likely results in the baby's brain modulating the pain, thereby causing the baby to feel less pain. When the mother picked the baby up and comforted her, the baby realized that the imminent danger was over. Realizing this, her brain then shut off the survival mode; her brain switched off its limbic system, which then stopped the stress reaction. In addition, her brain sent signals down to her spinal cord that helped to decrease the intensity of the pain signals being sent upward to her brain. **This is an example of how in response to changes in the environment and what you are thinking, the brain can modulate and affect the pain signals being sent to it from the spinal cord.**

This phenomenon occurs not just in babies, but also in adults. What you think about your pain has a direct effect on how you perceive your pain's intensity and how you behave toward it. What does this mean? You can modulate your pain sensations and how your brain and body react to them. You have power!

Our brains are constantly being flooded with all types of stimulation. It is your brain's job to interpret each stimulus and determine how to react to every sensation, including pain. The brain perceives and modulates every sensory stimulus that enters its chambers, even without your awareness. During the day, your brain is usually being bombarded with tons of sensations at once, but it can't react to everything at the same time. Therefore, your brain has evolved to focus and to figure out which sensations are important and deserve special attention.

MODULATION IN DAY-TO-DAY LIFE

Here's an example of brain modulation that we are sure you've encountered. Picture yourself with a friend in a crowded and noisy bar or restaurant. You have important issues to discuss. Even though you are surrounded by many other people having their own conversations, you are able to modulate what you listen to. You can block out all the other noises and focus on your friend's voice. However, if your friend goes to the restroom and leaves you alone, suddenly you hear all of the other conversations that you've been able to block out. It's not as though those conversations suddenly started—they were there the entire time. If you want to, you can listen, one at a time, to all the conversations that surround your table and then focus on the one that has the juiciest story and block out all the others. Well, the same kind of modulation happens with pain.

Take Advantage of Your Ability to Modulate!

So, how can you take advantage of this natural ability you're born with to modulate your sensations and your pain? **If you focus most of your attention on your pain, your brain will actually perceive more pain.** If pain is the most overwhelming stimulus entering your brain, your brain will actually amplify the pain volume and you will feel your pain more intensely. It's as though the brain must fill a certain stimulation quota. As we mentioned before, our brains crave stimulation. If you let the most important stimulation going to your brain be your pain, pain will preside as your president! Don't let this happen. Remember, impeachment is always an option.

Many people in pain don't even realize they are actually focusing their brain's attention on their pain. By simply staying at home (or worse, in bed) and not interacting with other people or not doing chores or not reading the newspaper, you are reducing the use of your other senses and are actually focusing your brain's attention on your pain. This is especially true at bedtime. Many persons-in-pain describe a worsening of their pain at bedtime. One possible explanation for this increase in pain is the need for your brain to be stimulated. At bedtime, it is dark and quiet; there's no visual or auditory stimulus. The only strong stimulus reaching your brain is your pain. Therefore, your brain turns up the volume to fill its sensation void.

Go Ahead and Be Driven to Distraction

Your brain craves stimulation. You can take advantage of this scientific fact to reduce your pain through distraction. That's right. It sounds simple, but it works! In fact, distraction is a true psychological technique that pain psychologists teach their patients. Fortunately, you generally don't need to spend good money to have someone teach you this technique. It's based on a simple fact: **If you keep your brain occupied with other sensations or thoughts, you will feel less pain.**

Did you ever notice that when you are involved in other activities (such as playing with your children or grandchildren, or watching a great ball game or movie) you feel less pain? You've been using the psychological technique of distraction without even realizing it. Try to remember to use distraction regularly every day to literally take your mind off your pain. The distraction can be almost anything, so find something that works and go with it! See table 15.1 for distraction techniques that are especially helpful at bedtime.

Table 15.1 Bedtime Distraction Techniques to Reduce Your Pain

- Read a book or magazine
- Write In a journal (not focused on your pain!)
- Listen to a meditation tape/CD
- Crochet/knit a present for a family memeber, friend, or yourself
- Sex—the ancient time-tested distraction technique!

CHAPTER 16

Laboratory Tests for Chronic Pain
(A Cautionary Tale)

Technology can help determine the problem

but not the processes of pain conditions.

No Easy Test for Chronic Pain

Most people today want to believe there is always a quick fix to their problems, including medical issues. And luckily for most of our medical problems, doctors can often quickly perform a medical test, whether it is a blood test or a radiological test, to find out what is wrong with us and then prescribe a medicine or send us to a surgeon to rid us of our symptoms. With chronic pain, it's usually not that simple.

TECHNOLOGY CAN HELP, SOMETIMES

Fortunately, we live in an age of miraculous technologies. Just think of all the cool new toys that weren't even imaginable when most of us were born or even in our teens—laptop computers the size of small briefcases, the ability to receive driving directions in our cars from a satellite, and the Internet revolution that allows us to get information about anything within a second (even if that information is wrong). Truly unbelievable!

In medicine, too, technology has revolutionized how doctors evaluate and treat their patients. Technology has helped us better understand the workings of both healthy bodies and those afflicted by disease. Machines such as computer-aided tomography (CT) scanners and magnetic resonance imaging (MRI) scanners allow doctors to visualize details of our innards and find cancers, blood clots, and tiny strokes. With each new generation of X-ray–like imaging machines, more and more detail is seen of the human body, which can be a great tool. However, we often forget that even though we can see more detail, doctors often do not understand the significance of these new findings. Frequently, doctors interpret these newfound results to reflect a disease state, only to find out later that what they observed was perfectly normal.

BEWARE OF TESTS THAT "SHOW YOU WHERE YOUR PAIN IS"

Although CT scanners, MRI machines, and other technologies have greatly helped doctors and many of their patients with lots of illnesses, the unfortunate truth is that these miraculous machines cannot help to locate the source of most cases of chronic pain. Such machines can sometimes help to identify the source of acute pain, but more often than not they are useless when it comes to helping us better understand chronic pain. **Both patients and physicians must realize that no machine or laboratory test can absolutely identify the source of chronic pain; nor can it measure the amount of pain felt by an individual.** Pain is a complex interaction of sensation and emotion, nerves and soft tissues, chemicals and electricity that just cannot be found or measured by any one test.

True Story of a New Technology Test Gone Bad

Here is a true example, a very sad story, of how a new type of test affected a doctor's decision in an unfortunate way. Back when MRI machines were first becoming available in U.S. medical centers (when we were in medical school) medical students were used as MRI guinea pigs. One unfortunate medical student—with no symptoms of disease—had MRI pictures taken of his brain. When the results came in, the radiologist noticed an unusual, never-before-seen tumor at the base of his brain. The neurosurgeon assumed this tumor to be cancerous and scheduled an emergency surgery to remove it. After surgery, the poor student was left with severe brain damage, never to become a doctor. To make matters worse, it was discovered that the tumor was benign. And several years later, it became known that the abnormal brain growth that the student had is not uncommon in normal brains and that these tumors don't grow. This medical student could have lived a normal life without the surgery. The take-home lesson here is to make sure your doctor fully understands any results from laboratory tests and how these results relate to your pain.

243

DON'T DIAGNOSE BY ONE TEST

It would therefore be foolhardy to expect that a machine that measures one single aspect of biologic function or takes a picture of a bodily structure can find the source of chronic pain. Just as it is foolish for a surgeon to perform exploratory surgery on a patient to find his or her pain, it is foolish for a doctor to order a laboratory test to find the pain. As one famous pain authority and neurosurgeon, Dr. John D. Loeser (one of our wisest pain management teachers and colleagues), has taught for many decades, "If a surgeon does surgery to try to find the pain of his patient, it will never be found."

TEST TO RULE OUT WHAT YOU DO NOT HAVE

When using laboratory tests, the rules for chronic pain diagnosis and treatment are very different compared to most other medical conditions. You must alter your expectations and your doctors must change their practices when it comes to diagnosing and treating chronic pain. You must not expect a laboratory test to show precisely where the pain is and why it is causing you so much unpleasantness and suffering; and your doctors must learn not to treat the test result, but to treat you, the entire patient.

Lab Tests Frequently Ordered by Doctors for Chronic Pain

Table 16.1 lists the types of lab tests that doctors frequently order in an effort to diagnose a patient's chronic pain. These tests are divided into two groups: radiological tests and electrophysiological studies.

WHAT DO THE DIFFERENT TESTS TELL US?

Radiological tests take pictures of different body parts to help identify any abnormalities that wouldn't be apparent just by looking at a person. These tests can tell us many things, including whether bones are broken; whether your internal organs, such as your liver, lungs, or kidneys, have abnormal growths or tumors; if soft tissues (muscles, ligaments, and tendons) are torn or inflamed; or if spinal discs are bulging.

Electrophysiological studies measure different electrical abilities of nerves. This helps to determine whether those peripheral nerves (that we learned are so important in pain signaling) are doing their job correctly. Remember, however, that even when these tests reveal an abnormality, it doesn't necessarily mean that this is the source of your pain.

Table 16.1: Radiological Tests and Electrophysical Sudies	
TYPES OF RADIOLOGICAL TESTS	**TYPES OF ELECTROPHYSIOLOGICAL STUDIES**
• X-ray • CT scan • MRI • Ultrasound • Myelogram • Bone scan	• Nerve conduction tests • Electromyography • Quantitative Sensory Testing

WHAT THESE TESTS CANNOT DETECT: REAL PAIN

What's more important than what these tests can tell us is what they cannot tell us. After all, many patients with chronic pain will have completely normal test results. Unfortunately, as you've already learned, doctors may misinterpret the fact that all your tests are normal. They may tell you (and your insurance company and workers' compensation board) that because all of the tests are normal, either the pain is psychogenic or you are malingering. When they say this, they are wrong 99.999 percent of the time. Having normal test results in no way means the pain is not real. Most often, normal lab tests in patients with chronic pain mean only that we lack the ability, even today, to detect important bodily functions that may look normal, but that cause pain. See Table 16.2 for a list of some specific things that laboratory tests cannot do.

Table 16.2: What Lab Tests Cannot Do

TYPES OF RADIOLOGICAL TESTS

We cannot measure how well the parts of your nervous system are working:

- We cannot assess whether all the parts of your nervous system are connected and communicating properly with one another.
- We cannot measure changes of your nervous system's natural chemical neurotransmitters, which are, as you have learned, the main way nerves communicate.

We cannot detect how well your musculoskeletal system is working:

- We have no laboratory test that can truly assess if your muscles are in spasm or if your ligaments and tendons have lost some of their elasticity.

CONCLUSION: PROCEED FROM TESTS WITH CAUTION

Though modern technology can rapidly advance research and save countless lives, it should not be blindly trusted. In the case of pain medicine, we still lack the ability to measure most of the processes responsible for your pain. For this reason, it is crucial that you and your doctor proceed with caution when reviewing results of any laboratory test, and consider the findings as only one tiny piece of an important whole: you.

CHAPTER 17

Stress Affects Your Pain, And It's Real

How you perceive your pain affects

how much you experience it.

Your Pain May Cause Psychological Problems—But Not Vice Versa!

To this day, we still unfortunately read articles in well-respected medical journals and textbooks that claim certain pain conditions are caused by psychological disorders. These arguments are mistakenly based on the fact that medical tests on many persons-in-pain reveal no abnormalities and that people with these conditions tend to suffer from psychological disorders. This type of illogical, ignorant thinking assumes that many chronic pain conditions are purely psychological in nature and, therefore, should be considered psychogenic pain.

The fact is that most patients in chronic pain suffer from psychological problems caused by being in chronic pain, such as depression, anxiety, or post-traumatic stress disorder, regardless of the pain condition or the specific individual afflicted. **Hear us loud and clear: Psychological problems rarely cause the pain— rather they are the result of pain!**

(continued)

Stress Makes Pain Worse

Most often, people with chronic pain experience a worsening of their condition with physical and/or emotional stress. Unfortunately, this is another piece of information misused by uneducated doctors, insurance companies, and lawyers as evidence to suggest that the pain is psychological in nature. This assumption is just wrong! In this chapter, we will discuss some scientific evidence regarding why your pain worsens when you get stressed.

The Stress Reaction is Predictable

What happens when you get into an argument with friends, a family member, or a co-worker? If you're like most human beings, you get stressed. But being stressed is not only a feeling or psychological state of mind. Your body reacts physically, and actually goes into a very predictable stress mode referred to as the *stress reaction*. As you might guess, the stress reaction is a series of physical functions your body produces as a response to stress. It's an automatic, natural body reaction that gets turned on during all stressful situations. And this physiological reaction occurs in all animals. Therefore, like pain itself, there is a reason we have stress reactions, but when associated with chronic pain the stress reaction loses its sense of purpose.

ADRENALINE TURNS UP THE PAIN

Whenever we experience stress, the chemical epinephrine (also referred to as *adrenaline*) is released into our bloodstream and travels throughout our body, causing many physiological changes to take place. When adrenaline gets near our pain nerves, it results in a significant increase in the number of pain signals sent to your brain—especially if these nerves are injured or inflamed. In other words, the nerves responsible for signaling pain are super-sensitive to adrenaline and begin to send stronger signals, causing your pain to actually intensify.

Similarly, muscles that are stiff and in spasm also are super-sensitive to adrenaline. So, when they are exposed to adrenaline, they actually go into more spasm and cause more pain.

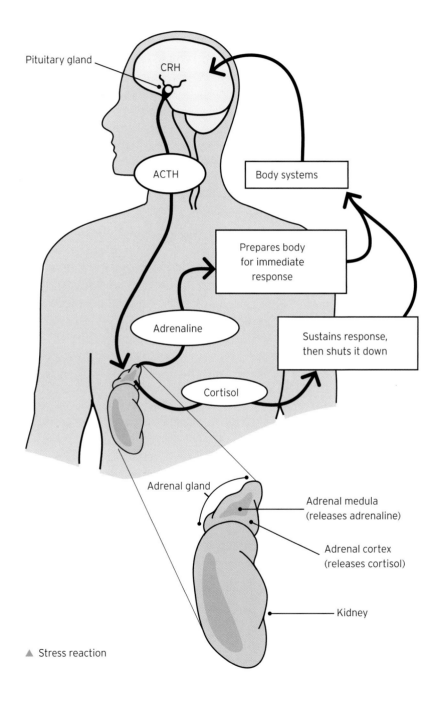

Pituitary gland

CRH

ACTH

Body systems

Prepares body for immediate response

Adrenaline

Sustains response, then shuts it down

Cortisol

Adrenal gland

Adrenal medula (releases adrenaline)

Adrenal cortex (releases cortisol)

Kidney

▲ Stress reaction

(Your Pain May Cause Psychological Problems–But Not Vice Versa! continued)

The take-home message is that **if you are depressed or anxious, you are completely normal!** It is very unfortunate when psychological complications of a person-in-pain are used against him or her. If a chronic pain patient is told that his or her pain is solely psychological in nature, it can only worsen the patient's pain, psychological state, and ultimately, his or her hope for successful treatment. This scenario can make you and your loved ones question your inner strength and diminish your chances for improvement. Please, don't let this happen to you!

249

A Fearful Memory: George's Story

George was in his fifties, a little overweight, and slightly worried about his health because his dad had died of a heart attack around the same age. One day, while eating a steak dinner (he likes it medium rare), he felt a sudden pain in his chest (on a scale of 1 to 10, the intensity was a 6). He was terrified that he was having a heart attack, and that thought made the pain even worse (a 10 out of 10). George's wife immediately drove him to the nearest emergency room. His pain remained very severe. He also began to breathe heavily, his heart began to race, and he was sweating profusely. Finally, he met with a doctor, and after some tests he learned that his pain was not a heart attack, but was caused by a stomach irritation (gastritis). He wasn't in danger of a heart attack after all. Within minutes, his pain rapidly eased to a 5 out of 10. He began to breathe regularly and his sweating stopped. What happened to relieve George's pain so quickly? (See "Frightening Memories Spark Pain.")

Your Memories and Pain

Another important and often-overlooked brain function that can have a huge impact on how you experience and respond to pain is your memory of it.

What does your pain mean to you? Think about this for a while, because it can be extremely important. How your brain and your body react to pain depends on what your pain reminds you of. If it reminds you of the nightmarish accident that caused your pain, your body will react in one way (stress!). If your pain reminds you of your glory days as a football quarterback, you'll probably react differently to your pain (glory days!).

MUSCLES ALSO REMEMBER PAIN

Although some memories can be so painful that they have been relegated to your subconscious, your body may still remember them. Sometimes something called *muscle memory* can occur: Your muscles "remember" the injury or a bad thing that happened, and will therefore respond in a different way than they did prior to the incident and formation of that memory. Quite often, when muscle memory is part of the pain problem, muscles can go into a constant state of tightness and spasm, exacerbating the pain.

Memories associated with pain can have very different effects. For some people they trigger the stress reaction, while for others they cause a calming or reassuring response. Therefore, your past experiences and memories can be a powerful weapon that you can use for or against the process of alleviating your pain. And all of this happens on a subconscious—or even unconscious—level, as various regions of the brain are turned either "on" or "off."

FRIGHTENING MEMORIES SPARK PAIN

In our sidebar, George originally felt his "heart" pain; he had a memory of his dad clutching his chest in pain and having a serious heart attack. When George first experienced his own pain, the memory of his dad came back to him and the stress reaction immediately turned on, causing his pain to amplify and his breathing and heart rate to increase, and causing him to sweat profusely.

What happened when the doctor told him it wasn't a heart attack? George was literally relieved. His brain turned off the stress reaction and voilà, his pain was instantly alleviated, his heart stopped racing, his breathing normalized, and he stopped sweating.

The doctor gave him some advice about treating his gastritis and about proper eating habits, and sent George on his way. The next time George experienced the same pain, it was frightening and it hurt; but because he knew it wasn't a heart attack, he was not as frightened, the pain didn't get worse, his heart didn't race and his breathing did not become heavy. And after ten minutes, the pain diminished.

How Your Brain Labels Pain

George's brain labeled the pain "bad pain," meaning "this pain is being caused by something that could do some serious damage to me!" However, when he found out the pain was from stomach acid and that it couldn't kill him, his brain immediately relabeled the pain as "not-bad pain." So, you see, **how you label your pain has a dramatic impact on how you feel pain and how your body reacts to it.**

The place in the brain where this labeling occurs is called the sensory cortex. "Bad pain" warns us that our body has been damaged or is about to be injured. So, what is "not-bad pain"? (Notice that we didn't call it "good" pain because that's kind of an oxymoron in our minds.) Think of it as training for a marathon. To condition their bodies, athletes must push themselves to their physical limits. It's like that old saying, "No pain, no gain"; when in training, athletes feel pain, but this doesn't stop them from accomplishing their goals. How you label your pain has a huge effect on how you experience it. Because this is very important, we're going to repeat it: **How you label your pain has a huge effect on how you experience your pain.**

Let's compare a pain if you label it as "bad" versus "not bad."

"BAD PAIN" GOES LIMBIC

If you and your brain label your pain as "bad, where do you think the pain signal travels in your brain? Yup, you guessed it; the pain signal goes right to the limbic system. As we mentioned before, the limbic system consists of some of the oldest of the brain's structures—all animals have a limbic system. The limbic system plays an important role in our survival and is involved in all of our basic drives: hunger, thirst, pain, and sex.

Pain Alert!

Be Careful What You Think!
If your back pain is making you think, "My disc may pop at any second, squeeze my spinal cord, and then maybe even paralyze me" (which is highly unlikely to occur, by the way), you are labeling your pain as "bad pain." If you think the headaches you are having may be due to a brain tumor when they're actually migraine headaches, you are labeling your pain as "bad pain" and will experience all the nasty stuff that comes along with this label. Just thinking that your pain means scary, bad things are happening to you will have a bad effect on your pain and your body! But remember that chronic pain happens after the acute injury has healed, so you have to keep reminding yourself (and your brain) that this pain you are feeling does not mean damage has been done to your body.

The limbic system is considered part of the autonomic nervous system (ANS) and is responsible for the stress reaction. In a stressful situation, the ANS causes stress hormones (one of the most important being adrenalin) to be released from the pituitary gland within the brain. Adrenalin flowing through our blood then heightens our awareness of our environment and increases our heart and breathing rates (like a super-rush of caffeine from a triple-shot espresso). Importantly, when the brain's limbic system is turned on, it sends pain-modulating signals down to the pain region of the spinal cord (remember the Gate Control Theory we discussed in chapter 15).

At first, during the initial phases of the stress reaction, this signal from the brain actually causes a reduction in the pain signal. This process is termed *stress analgesia* and can actually be quite effective in blocking you from feeling any pain.

"FIGHT OR FLIGHT" NUMBS THE PAIN INITIALLY

Why would nature want us to initially stop the pain we are feeling under stress? Well, the reaction is actually quite conducive to survival. Consider this: You've just been injured badly (say, during a battle) and you are still in the situation that can cause you further bodily harm (your enemy is now trying to kill you). To survive, you need to either fight or run away (the fight or flight phenomenon). But if you actually felt the horrible pain caused by your injuries, you'd feel like crawling into a ball, crying, and giving up hope—and surely you'd have no chance of survival! You'd be a goner for sure. But if you don't feel the pain, perhaps you have a chance of survival. We have been designed to increase our chance of survival by not feeling the true amount of pain from our injuries under stress.

Examples of stress analgesia occur all the time. Consider the soldier whose limb was badly damaged after a bomb exploded and yet is able to find his fellow injured soldiers and drag them to safety; or the all-star running back who fractures a bone in the first quarter, but plays the entire game with minimal pain because it's the Super Bowl and he wants that ring. Evolution in action!

CHRONIC STRESS IS A SOURCE OF REAL PAIN

However, the great pain-reducing power of the stress reaction is very short-lived. If you feel stressed for too long (several days), your limbic system begins to turn against you. Not only do you lose the pain-relieving effects you initially experienced, but also the physical stress of pain now actually makes matters worse. Stress becomes your enemy.

When chronic pain leads to persistent activation of the stress reaction, bad things start to happen. The brain's limbic system changes its signals to the spinal cord from a pain reducing effect (-) to a pain amplification effect (+). You therefore begin to feel more pain. Additionally, chronic stress can weaken the immune system; after being "on alert" for long periods of time your body becomes tired and weakened. Chronic stress also has been shown to increase the risk of heart disease, diabetes, depression, and anxiety disorders. Therefore, by continually labeling your chronic pain as "bad," you actually turn up the pain volume and cause other nasty stuff to happen to your body, such as making you more prone to depression, anxiety, heart disease, diabetes, and even catching colds and the flu!

"NOT-BAD" PAIN PROVIDES NATURAL PAIN RELIEF

Now let's examine the opposite. What happens to the pain signal after it reaches your brain and you label it as "not-bad" pain, meaning that you do not believe this pain means damage or danger to your body? **If you feel as though the pain you are experiencing (even if it is very severe) does not represent an underlying threat to your body, the nasty limbic system is turned "off" and no stress reaction occurs.** That's right, no stress reaction occurs! (Doesn't that feel good already?)

And there's more good news! If you label the pain as "not bad," the pain signal travels to another primitive and important brain area, the periaqueductal gray (PAG). The PAG is where scientists have actually found natural opiate (morphine-like) substances called *endorphins*. When you label the pain as "not-bad," the pain signal travels from the brain's sensory cortex to the PAG, instead of the limbic system, where your pain would have been amplified, and the reverse happens! When the PAG is turned on, it releases those natural endorphins in your brain, causing you to feel less pain, as though you took a painkiller. Free medicine! Additionally, when the PAG is turned on, it sends pain-relieving signals to the pain's spinal cord gate, reducing the pain signals that are going up to your brain—another way you will feel less pain.

So, by simply labeling your chronic pain as "not-bad," you can naturally decrease your pain level by releasing your own organic painkillers deep within your brain, and also reduce the amount of pain being transmitted from your spinal cord to your brain. Way cool!

253

Learn How to Manage Your Stress

It is clear that the stress response is biological, not psychological. These bodily reactions are the reason why stress management tools are often recommended to treat chronic pain patients. Stress management techniques, such as biofeedback and imagery (see chapter 11), can take time to learn, but if you put effort into practicing them they can provide significant pain relief—what's more, they are available to you 24/7, at no cost, and without side effects.

A LITTLE MIND TRAINING GOES A LONG WAY

You can see why most pain clinics and pain psychologists put a lot of time and effort into teaching their patients how to label their pain as "not-bad." Although your pain may be severe and horrible, it doesn't mean that every time you feel it, you are damaging your body. Remember: Pain doesn't always mean harm.

You need to understand, though, that your brain initially labels all pain as "bad pain"—and why shouldn't it? After all, 99.99 percent of the time, the pain you experience is "bad pain." Chronic pain is an unfortunate anomaly; it feels just like pain that comes with an injury, even though there isn't any ongoing damage. Therefore, people living with chronic pain must be proactive in training their brain to relabel the pain they feel.

Pain psychologists and physical therapists can help you train your brain by using certain tricks, or you can teach yourself. It's like training an old dog (a very smart one, mind you!): Whenever you feel your chronic pain, make a point of consciously thinking that the pain you are feeling is "not-bad" pain and does not mean damage is being done to you. Another way you can train your brain is by doing things that trigger your chronic pain (we know, it doesn't sound fun, but it will help!). By doing the activities that elicit your pain and by showing your brain that no damage was done, your brain eventually understands and learns that indeed this is not damaging, "bad pain."

Remember: You can do it! It takes daily practice to make your brain realize that your chronic pain is not "bad pain," but we know for sure that relabeling of your pain is worth it.

The Stress Reaction and Guarding
GUARDING IS A BIG PROBLEM IN CHRONIC PAIN

Your brain cannot differentiate between acute pain and chronic pain. When you feel pain after an injury has already healed (as in the case of chronic pain), the stress reaction and innate desire to guard your body become your enemy. **You have to consciously reteach your brain that the stress reaction and guarding are in the wrong place at the wrong time.** The stress reaction that causes you to chronically guard and protect your hurting body part is also likely to be responsible for some additional pain.

Another observation frequently made of persons-in-pain is that the guarding of the painful body part causes other body regions to develop painful problems due to either overuse or disuse. For instance, if a patient with leg pain limps so that he or she will favor the right leg, eventually the patient's left leg, hip, and lower back will develop tight and spastic muscles (myofascial dysfunction) because they are being overused. These muscles in spasm will cause new areas of pain.

How to Apply Lessons Learned from the Astronauts and Rats

Consider the following example of what happens if you don't use your muscles and bones regularly. NASA engineers learned a lesson during the early days of space flight. They noticed that following several days in space, where there is no gravity and astronauts move their bodies minimally, rapid musculoskeletal changes occurred from lack of normal use. Astronauts were coming home with spasms and atrophy (shrinkage) of their muscles, shortening and loss of elasticity of tendons and ligaments, and loss of bone density—all things that can happen to chronic pain patients if they don't move their body normally. To prevent these bodily changes from occurring, NASA now requires a daily exercise routine for all astronauts during space flight.

Recently, scientists have demonstrated similar findings in rats. When a rat is restrained from using a leg (by wearing a cast on the leg, though the leg is not injured at all), changes occur in the rat's spinal cord. And what's fascinating (at least to us) is that these changes in the rat's spinal cord are similar to changes observed after the rat's leg has had a painful nerve injury. Thus, chemical and nerve changes occur in your spinal cord (and we have to assume in your brain too) just because you stop using your arm, leg, or back normally!

These examples should show that when you do not actively use your body in a normal way, things stop working as they normally would—and all of these changes can cause even more pain. Therefore, it is crucial that you take action to prevent such changes!

CONCLUSION: UNDERSTANDING LEADS TO LOWER STRESS AND LESS PAIN

As you have read, the stress reaction is a normal part of living. It plays a very important and vital role in our survival. But when it's associated with chronic pain, it can cause you further problems. The good news is that you can make huge improvements in your chronic pain just by understanding the stress reaction and making some changes in how you react to stress.

Get the Facts: Immobilization Leads to Pain

By not moving a body part, the following problems of "disuse" can occur:

- Muscle atrophy (shrinkage), causing weakness
- Muscle tightness and spasm (myofascial dysfunction), causing pain
- Shortening and loss of the normal elasticity of tendons and ligaments, causing loss of movement and pain with movement
- Brittle bones, causing potential fractures

255

Appendix: Helpful Web Sites

Patient information Web sites:

- Pain education for health care providers (www.painedu.org)
- Pain education for patients (www.painaction.com)
- National Pain Foundation (www.nationalpainfoundation.org)
- American Pain Foundation (www.painfoundation.org)
- Reflex Sympathetic Dystrophy Syndrome Association (www.rsdsa.org)
- The Neuropathy Association (www.neuropathy.org)
- Fibromyalgia (www.fmaware.org)
- American Chronic Pain Association (www.theacpa.org)
- Financial Assistance Resource Guide (www.rsdsa.org/4/resources/out_work/in_pain_intro.html)

Pain medical societies:

- American Pain Society (www.ampainsoc.org)
- American Academy of Pain Medicine (www.painmed.org)
- American Academy of Pain Management (www.aapainmanage.org)

Headache medical societies:

- International Headache Society (www.i-h-s.org)
- American Headache Society (www.americanheadachesociety.org)

Patient information headache Web sites:

- American Headache Society Committee for Headache Education (www.achenet.org)
- Headache education for patients (www.painaction.com)
- American Academy of Neurology (www.thebrainmatters.org)
- National Institutes of Health (www.nlm.nih.gov/medlineplus/headache.html)
- National Headache Foundation (www.headaches.org)

Acknowledgments

The authors would like to acknowledge and thank Caitlin Shure for her assistance and the team at Fair Winds Press, especially Laura Smith, Tiffany Hill, and Jill Alexander, for making this book possible. We would also like to thank all of our teachers and colleagues, with whom we have been lucky to work beside and learn from, including some of the great minds and clinicians in pain management; thank you for sharing your knowledge and friendship.

DR. CHARLES ARGOFF

I would like to thank my long-time friend, Brad Galer, for co-writing this book and always being there to discuss professional projects and personal developments. I thank my parents, Allen and Renee Argoff, for teaching me not only the value of hard work and dedication, but also the value of compassion and caring for all people. I'd like to thank my wife, Patty, for her boundless love and never-ending patience and support. Lastly, I thank my children, David, Melanie, and Emily, each of whom is amazing and whom I love dearly.

DR. BRAD GALER

I would like to thank my long-time friend, Charles Argoff, for co-writing this book and for the hundreds of other achievements we have made together. My parents, Marilyn and Larry Galer, instilled in me the importance of pursuing dreams and helping others. I would also like to thank my loving wife, Lele, who has always stood beside me and supported all the endeavors I have dreamed and pursued; and my sons, Alex, Peter, and Simon, who are marvelously unique and wonderful: You make me proud every day.

About the Authors

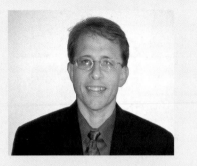

CHARLES E. ARGOFF, M.D.

Dr. Argoff is professor of neurology at Albany Medical College (NY) and director of the Comprehensive Pain Center at Albany Medical Center (NY). He received his medical degree from Northwestern University's Feinberg School of Medicine in Chicago, and completed an internship in the Department of Medicine and a residency in the Department of Neurology at the State University of New York in Stony Brook, and a fellowship in developmental and metabolic neurology at the National Institutes of Health/National Institute of Neurological Disorders and Stroke.

Dr. Argoff is a member of the International Association for the Study of Pain, the American Academy of Pain Medicine, and the American Academy of Neurology, among other professional organizations. He serves on the editorial board of the *Clinical Journal of Pain* and as a reviewer for the *Journal of Pain, Brain, JAMA, Archives of Physical Medicine* and *Rehabilitation, Journal of Musculoskeletal Pain, Journal of Pain and Symptom Management,* and *Clinical Journal of Pain*. He is co-editor of the Neuropathic Pain Section of *Pain Medicine.*

Dr. Argoff has served as a guest editor for and published articles in the *Clinical Journal of Pain and Current Pain and Headache Reports*, among other peer-reviewed journals. He has written on many types of pain, including myofascial pain, spinal and radicular pain, and neuropathic pain. He has written on such treatments as topical analgesics, interventional pain management, botulinum toxins, and oral analgesics, and has contributed many book chapters as well. Dr. Argoff had an active role in the development of the diabetic peripheral neuropathic pain guidelines published in *Mayo Clinic Proceedings*, and he has contributed to other published neuropathic pain treatment guidelines. He is one of the editors of the recently published textbook Raj's Practical *Management of Pain*, Fourth Edition. He also recently published the third edition of *Pain Management Secrets*.

He lives with his wife, Patty, and their three wonderful children, David, Melanie and Emily, in Loudonville, New York.

BRADLEY S. GALER, M.D.

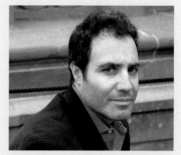

Dr. Galer obtained his B.A. in biology-psychology from Wesleyan University (CT) and his M.D. from Albert Einstein College of Medicine (NY). He completed a neurology residency at Albert Einstein, where he was chief resident, and then two pain fellowships, at Memorial Sloane-Kettering (NY) and the University of California at San Francisco. He has been an assistant professor at the University of Washington (Seattle) and associate professor at Albert Einstein, where he cared for patients, performed clinical research, and taught. In 2000, he joined Endo Pharmaceuticals as senior medical officer. Currently, he is president of the Pain Group of Nuvo Research.

Dr. Galer is a founding member and former chair of the Pain Medicine Section of the American Academy of Neurology, as well as a member of the Initiative on Methods, Measurement, and Pain Assessment in Clinical Trials, a collaboration between pharma, the U.S. Food and Drug Administration, the National Institutes of Health, academia, and patient advocacy groups. He has published more than 200 articles and book chapters, as well as lectured worldwide. He has co-authored the gold-standard book *Clinical Guide to Neuropathic Pain*, is the founding editor-in-chief of the journal *Current Pain and Headache Reports*, and is on the Editorial Board of *The Clinical Journal of Pain*. He was awarded Best Doctor in America and honored by the Neuropathy Association for his work in neuropathic pain. He is on the Board of Directors for the Reflex Sympathetic Dystrophy Syndrome Association. He is founder of Galer Estate Vineyard & Winery located in the Brandywine Valley of Pennsylvania. He is married to his college sweetheart, Lele, and has three great kids: Alex, Peter, and Simon.

Index

for migraines, 96
for neck pain, 34
rebound headache syndrome and, 111
for rheumatoid arthritis, 62
craniosacral therapy
for back pain, 20
for migraines, 99
for neck pain, 37
cryoanalgesia, 191
CT scans, 245–246
cyclobenzaprine (Flexeril), 39
for fibromyalgia, 121
cyclooxygenase (COX), 48. *See also* COX-1 inhibitors; COX-2 inhibitors
Cymbalta (duloxetine)
for back pain, 17
for cancer pain, 141
diabetic painful neuropathy and, 168
for fibromyalgia, 121, 122
for osteoarthritis, 49
for postherpetic neuralgia, 74
for rheumatoid arthritis, 63
side effects, 122

D
Dantrium (dantrolene), 39
dantrolene (Dantrium), 39
deep brain stimulation, 192
Demerol (meperidine), for cancer pain, 141
Depakote (divalproex sodium/volproic acid)
for migraines, 97, 165
side effects, 144, 164
depression. *See also* tricyclic antidepressants (TCAs)
back pain and, 21
medical treatments, 203

nonmedication-based treatments, 204–207
signs of, 201
desensitization, 197–198
desipramine. *See* tricyclic antidepressants (TCAs)
desvenlafaxine (Pristiq), for cancer pain, 141
dextromethorphan, for cancer pain, 143
diabetic neuropathy. *See* painful polyneuropathy/diabetic neuropathy
diabetic painful neuropathy (DPN), 168
diabetic peripheral neuropathic pain (DPNP), 167
diagnostic nerve blocks, 183
diclofenac, 75
Dilantin (phenytoin)
for cancer pain, 142
side effects, 144, 164
disc, slipped or bulged, 25, 28
disease-modifying antirheumatic drugs. *See* DMARDS
divalproex sodium (Depakote)
for migraines, 97, 165
side effects, 144, 164
DMARDS (disease-modifying antirheumatic drugs)
for back pain, 27
for osteoarthritis, 44
for rheumatoid arthritis, 60–62
doctors, incorrect assumptions about pain, 224–225
dry-needling, 19, 36, 181
duloxetine (Cymbalta)
for back pain, 17
for cancer pain, 141
diabetic painful neuropathy and, 168

for fibromyalgia, 121, 122
for osteoarthritis, 49
for postherpetic neuralgia, 74
for rheumatoid arthritis, 63
side effects, 122
Dysport, 19, 37

E
Effexor (venlafaxaine)
about, 167
for cancer pain, 141
electrical stumulation, 191–192
electromyogram (EMG)
cautions, 79, 245–246
for diagnosing back pain, 25
for diagnosing neck pain, 39
electrophysiological tests, 244–246
eletriptan (Relpax), for migraines, 95
emotional stress. *See* stress; stress management
Enbrel (etanercept)
for back pain, 27
for rheumatoid arthritis, 62
endorphins, 253
Entereg (alvimopan), for cancer pain, 142
epidural steroid injections (ESI), 187–188
episodic tension-types headaches, 108
ergotamines, rebound headache syndrome and, 111
escitalopram (Lexapro), for cancer pain, 141
etanercept (Enbrel)
for back pain, 27
for rheumatoid arthritis, 62
etoricoxbib (Arcoxia), 161
excitation, of neurotransmitters, 233